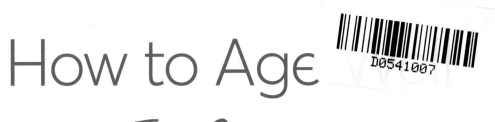

How to Age Well
The Secrets

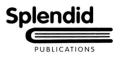

Splendid
PUBLICATIONS

How To Age Well
The Secrets

Anthea Turner

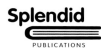

Splendid Publications Ltd,
1 Maple Place,
London W1T 4BB

www.splendidpublications.co.uk

British Library Cataloguing in Publication Data is available from The British Library

ISBN: 978-1-909109-81-0

Designed by Chris Fulcher

Printed and bound by Swallowtail Print, Drayton Industrial Park, Norwich NR8 6RL

Commissioned by Shoba Ware

How to Age Well
The Secrets

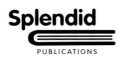

Splendid
PUBLICATIONS

ANTHEA TURNER

Old age ain't no place for sissies

—— Bette Davis ——

CONTENTS

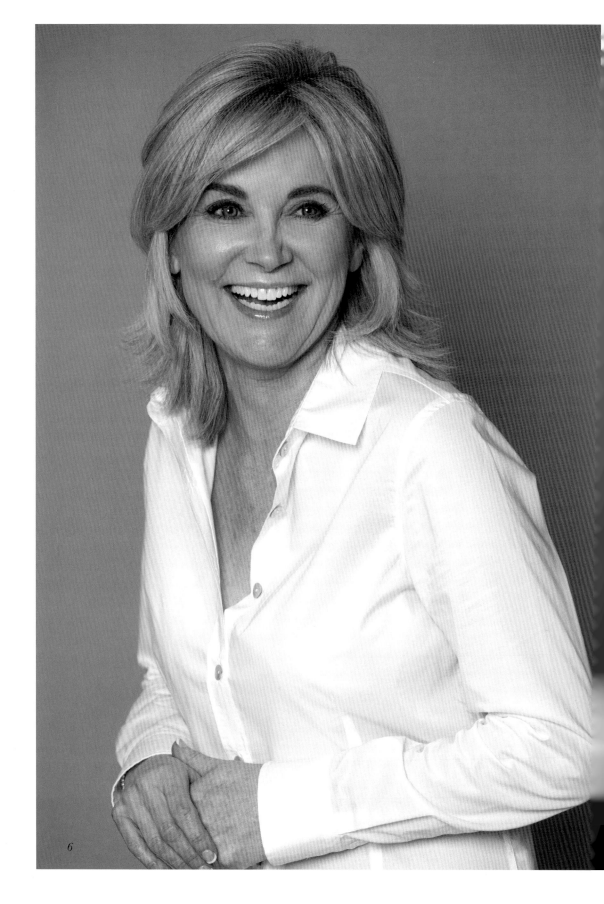

INTRODUCTION

— by Anthea Turner —

I HAVE always believed the secret to looking young is not in a pot of cream but in your attitude. Jump in the sea on a sunny day or in a perfect puddle in the rain and you will see what I mean. If you have lost your exuberance for life it will show on your face and in your body, but this book is set to change all that, not only by helping you get the positive mental attitude you need, but by sharing some of my favourite tips, tricks, hacks and habits to help you look and feel youthful again.

I'm guessing that if you've bought this book you've come to the conclusion you have more air miles behind you than in front, you've seen your mortality, stared it in the face and now are on a quest to enter what the Japanese call your 'second spring' with commitment and enthusiasm.

But what are the secrets to ageing well? How much is in your genes, environment, influences? What commitment will it take to look the way you want as you grow older? Is it too late to make a difference? Will I actually live longer; is that the point of ageing well? Whether the elixir of youth is in the mind, a jar of serum or a surgeon's knife, we all want to find it! Like me, you will have stood in front of the mirror scrutinising your face and body knowing the reflection looking back at you is the first sign of visible ageing: a few extra pounds, wrinkles, hair not the mane it once was…Skin still covers your body but there seems to be a little extra like a dress that needs taking in and if you're fair skinned what are those dark little marks?

Then, what's going on inside? The menopause, sexual and gynaecological changes, ageing organs, bones, muscles, joints. Then there's your state of mind, most likely related to your work life, significant relationship, children, family, friendships, finances, balance of pleasure and purpose.

Over the years, I have found myself looking closely at women I respected and admired, idly reading up on their lives, scanning for little nuggets of advice I could knit into my life.

I've subconsciously picked up books written by doctors, aesthetic surgeons, psychiatrists, thinkers, bloggers, lifestyle gurus, all professionals, as well as SAS soldiers, athletes and spiritual leaders, all the while searching for their secrets, making good use of the ones that work and discarding the gimmicks that don't….and now it's time to share those with you.

Don't get me wrong, I'm not talking cryogenics here but who, given the choice wants to grow prematurely old? One of the great gifts maturity gives you is a pin sharp sense of time. I can feel, smell and taste the next twenty-five years because the last twenty-five have gone like a shooting star.

So what have I done in this book to help you? The leg work. I've pored through books, spoken to experts looking for the workable tips tricks and 'secrets' that if you adopt will be significant in your desire to age well. Over the many years I've worked in television, I've been fortunate enough to work with so many talented people, experts in their field who have shared with me their advice and helpful tips. In *How to Age Well: The Secrets*, I'm sharing many of them with you.

I worked on this project with my friend and publisher Shoba Ware and our mutual friend Alison Webster, a fantastic photographer who has taken most of the images. (A big thank you to Eastwell Manor Champneys Hotel & Spa www.champneys.com/hotels/eastwell-manor who hosted many of our photoshoots.)

Through Covid19 restrictions, we relied on each other rather than a retinue of makeup artists, directors and stylists: it just goes to show what you can achieve yourself!

I don't expect you to read this book from cover to cover: it's a dip-in, dip-out guide to keep for when you need it. I hope you will find the expert advice provided by my amazing contributors - as well as my own tips - insightful and helpful. Enjoy!

Anthea

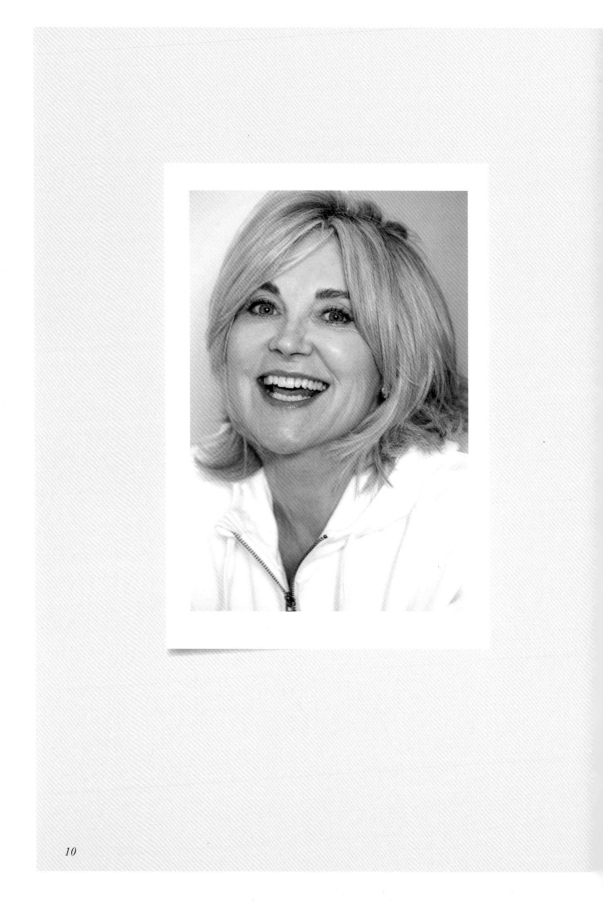

CHAPTER 1

—— The Menopause Challenge ——

BEFORE I started going through the menopause in my early fifties, I knew very little about the subject, practically nothing in fact apart from apparently your periods stopped and you had a few hot sweats. How wrong I was!

I don't remember hearing or reading much about the menopause in the media and I certainly don't remember my doctor talking about it, and saying, 'Oh by the way, how are your periods? We'd like to prepare you for menopause; you know we're here, these are the symptoms to look out for, just let us know.' That's because it simply didn't happen. It's so good that women – and men! – are talking more about this subject because it shouldn't be taboo. It's a natural part of the ageing process and how you deal with it can make all the difference to how you feel about yourself and life in general.

The only reason I had any conversations about my body clock was due to the fact that I was late to the party in wanting a baby. I was one of those women who was busy working and always saying, 'Oh I'll get round to it one day.' I also have throughout my life been a late developer. I didn't get *Blue Peter*, my big gig in television until I was thirty-two. Everything I've done has been late so I'm sort of used to being the last in and catching up.

***

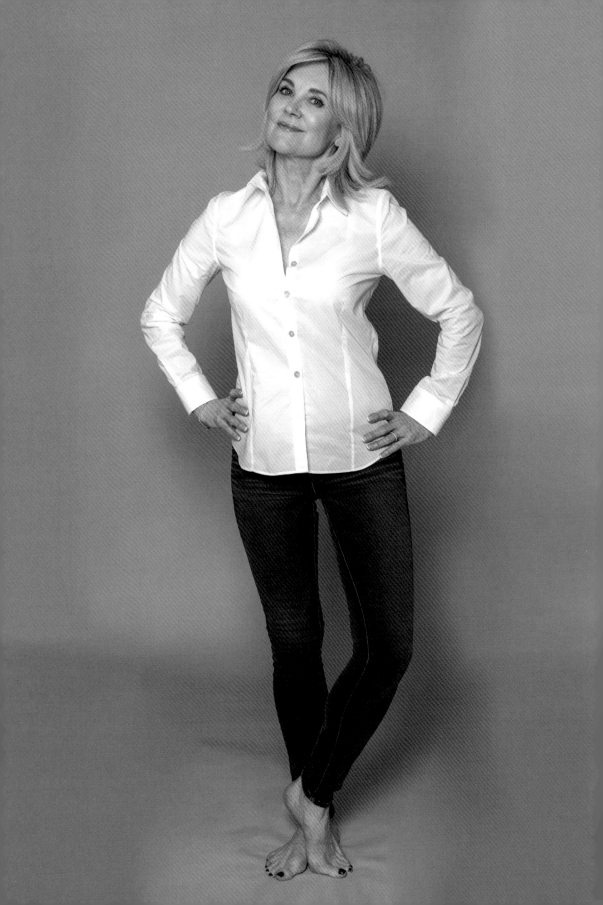

When I was thirty-eight, my ex-husband Grant Bovey and I met and my maternal instinct finally kicked in. I know some people grow up wanting a baby but it wasn't me. I also believed, it 'just happens' which is another thing nobody told me; it doesn't always 'just happen'.

In 1999, I started trying to get pregnant but things weren't happening naturally, and a gynaecologist I went to see said, 'Look, you haven't got time on your side and if I were you, I wouldn't mess around. I would go straight for IVF. You can't wait; your body clock is ticking pretty fast.' So that was probably the first time I started to really have proper conversations about my 'down belows.' But I don't remember the word menopause being used even then. It was all about, before you get too old, before your eggs stop.

As it turned out, it was quite a while before I hit menopause. My periods started going a bit 'funny' when I was fifty-one. It starts quite slowly where they're late or heavy or you miss one. And for all the problems I'd had with IVF (sadly, it didn't work for us), I'd always been fairly regular. That's when the first proper menopause conversations began for me and they weren't easy to have.

Once the perimenopause happens, you are embarrassed because this is the first real sign of age. This is your internal structure taking over now and saying, 'Girl, I know they weren't much good in the first place but now your reproductive opportunities are well and truly over.'

I'm generally a fit, healthy woman with loads of energy so the shock for me was I just didn't feel right and I couldn't put my finger on it. I wasn't feeling very well, not sexy. I was looking in the mirror feeling dull and sweaty. I couldn't quite get my head around what the problem was. You just don't feel the same - it's the weirdest, weirdest thing. And it's a shock and you're embarrassed and you don't really want to talk about it.

I did try and talk to my husband about it, but he wasn't interested. I even wrote him a letter, which I found years later when I moved. Unbeknown to me at the time, Grant had taken up with a twenty-four year-old so of course he wasn't interested in his sweaty, dull, wife's problems. In the letter I told him, I just want you to know what's happening. I said this is what's happening to my body and I'm so sorry but I'm just not being myself.

I felt that I was being miserable. I was struggling to be as active as I would normally be. Finally I went to see this lovely lady doctor at my local NHS practice. I sat down with her and burst into tears and said, 'I really don't know what is the matter with me. I've been here before and one of the other doctors gave me some tranquillisers but I really don't want to take them.' She listened carefully and when I'd finished told me, 'No, no, no, no, no. What you need is HRT.' Those magic tablets changed everything. For a while.

∗∗∗

I'm not so sure if HRT worked immediately, because the problem was I was going through a divorce which was painful. So, I was going through menopause, a divorce, moving house and death. I say death because divorce is a death; it's the death of the life of a marriage. But you're also going through the loss of your youth. And you're mourning both of those things.

I was also going through the humiliation of seeing it all played out in the media and seeing my husband with someone who represented who I used to be: fun, carefree, no responsibilities. I can stand back now and dissect it and understand, but at the time I was in a complete and utter visceral fog, which I had difficulty explaining to anyone.

We now know far more about menopause and HRT and it's not necessarily a one tablet fits all. While those tablets the GP helped me to begin with, the effects didn't last which goes to show you need to make sure you are on the right type of HRT for YOU. If you possibly can, see a GP who is a hormone specialist as they understand what best to prescribe for your particular symptoms. I remember arriving at an event I was presenting and thought, 'There's something not right with me.' In the hotel room getting changed, I absolutely fell apart; I simply couldn't get my act together. I was sweating. I could feel my head start to sweat and my face go red.

I hate using the term, 'pull yourself together' but that evening I had no choice but to do just that. I still don't know how I got through it and drove the two hours home afterwards. I knew I had to do something quickly to avoid that scenario ever happening again.

I was recommended an amazing menopause expert by the name of Dr Louise Newson, also known as The Menopause Doctor. She did blood tests to check my hormone levels and after an in-depth conversation about my symptoms and health history prescribed me everything my body needed accordingly. Within three weeks, I was breathing a huge sigh of relief and felt a lot closer to my old self.

"HRT is the gold standard menopause treatment: it corrects hormone deficiency, eases symptoms and protects future health – but too many women are unaware of its benefits, or worse still, are denied a prescription. It's a key reason why I founded both The Menopause Charity and my balance menopause app to campaign for, and provide, clear-evidenced based information on all things HRT and menopause. If you are suffering in silence, it's never too late to educate yourself and seek help so you can access treatment like HRT."

—— **Dr Louise Newson** ——

Dr Louise Newson is a leading menopause specialist. She is the founder of the free balance menopause support app www.balance-app.com and the founder of The Menopause Charity.

I'm now on body identical HRT – not to be confused with bioidentical – which is different. I use oestrogen gel, testosterone gel – yeah! – and take progesterone tablets and have no menopausal symptoms at all. I'm religious about taking my meds. I feel full of energy and optimistic and I find it helps control my weight. I'm not one for piling on the pounds easily but menopause changed all that. Yet another reason to stay on HRT!

HRT makes a difference to your skin, your hair, your demeanour; just about everything. A friend of mine who lectures on the subject says she can tell in a

Difficulty concentrating

Dizziness

Hair changes

Headache and migraines

Changes to taste and smell

Brain fog

Dry eyes

Mood swings

Dry mouth

Night sweats

Dental issues

Depression

Burning mouth

Anxiety

Breast tenderness

Heart disease

Heart palpitations

Breathing difficulties

Fatigue

Bladder infections

Vaginal dryness

Fertility issues

Vaginal irritation and itching

Loss of sex drive

Loss of confidence and self-esteem

Period changes

Altered skin sensation

Osteoporosis

Weight gain

Lack of motivation

Body odour

Hot flushes

Changes to nails

Muscle aches and pains

Skin changes

Joint pains

Sleep issues

Forgetfulness

THIRTY-EIGHT SYMPTOMS OF PERIMENOPAUSE AND MENOPAUSE

room of menopausal women the ones who are on HRT just by looking at them. Frankly I will stay on it for the rest of my life. There's no reason to come off it as far as I'm concerned.

I know I sound zealous about HRT and for me, it is the right thing. It works. But I also know that it's not suitable for everyone. If it's not for you, there are ways to cope with menopausal symptoms naturally which we'll explain in this chapter. I'm a great believer in eating well, exercising and mindfulness; all wonderful tools to help combat what every woman will go through in one way or another.

$$- \mathcal{A} -$$

When it comes to the menopause and all things hormonal, there is no one more qualified or knowledgeable than Consultant Gynaecologist and Director of Hormone Health, **Mr Nick Panay.** I won't list all his qualifications here, there are too many of them!

I was fortunate enough to meet Nick at a Wellbeing of Women (www. wellbeingofwomen.org.uk) discussion I was chairing in Birmingham in 2019 and he completely dispelled all the misconceptions I'd heard about hormone replacement therapy. By then I was already on HRT as Dr Louise Newson who was speaking at the event had prescribed it for me and changed my life but Nick in his calm and measured way, left me completely enlightened, confident I was on the right path.

As well as being one of the busiest doctors I know (see his biog for more) he is also one of the most generous in terms of his time in getting women the help they need when it comes to the challenge that is the menopause. Despite his hectic schedule, he agreed to answer some questions I know many of you want answers to when it comes to the menopause and the whole question of HRT:

WHY IS THERE STILL CONFUSION ABOUT TAKING HRT?

"IT has been a bit of a roller coaster ride. Some years back, hormone replacement therapy was considered as the universal panacea and women were rushing to be prescribed as there was this idea that there were no real risks, only an upside. Then came the initial findings of the World Health Initiative (WHI) trials, published in 2002, which wrongly claimed HRT had more negative than beneficial effects. Overnight, the use of HRT among women plummeted by about fifty per cent. There was an overreaction to those studies and too many women came off hormone therapy even if they weren't at risk. What we realised after the WHI is that if you use the wrong dose of HRT in the wrong age group, then there potentially could be some risks – small but significant. The average age of women in the study was sixty-three and women as old as seventy-nine were being given relative overdoses of hormone therapy. The other frustrating thing was when the data was originally released, they said it applied across all age groups but this wasn't the case.

Now we understand the problems with those studies in that hormone therapy wasn't properly individualised. If you appropriately individualise hormone therapy then you can maximise effectiveness and minimise risks.

HAS UPTAKE OF HRT INCREASED IN RECENT YEARS?

Yes, I definitely think it has and is improving still. There was certainly a legacy of fear after the WHI findings but now I believe we are on track to repair it. In terms of types of preparations of HRT we have moved on. We individualise hormone therapy much more and people and health care professionals are realising if you give the right preparation for the right indication to the right woman, there are hardly any side effects and it's hugely beneficial.

WHAT'S THE BEST WAY OF TAKING HRT?

Generally speaking, HRT is made up of oestrogen, progesterone and testosterone, although not all women have all three, depending on individual need. How you administer HRT is as important as the dosage itself. Oestrogen can be prescribed in tablet form but we now prefer to prescribe it in the form of a patch, gel or spray as there's no increased risk of clotting when used through the skin. At the moment there are no good data to say that oestrogen through the skin is any different in terms of safety for the breast, compared to oral oestrogen. However, what people often don't realise is that progesterone is equally as important as oestrogen and if we use a natural progesterone then it's better from the breast perspective. We don't need to routinely use synthetic types of progesterone or progestogens as we used to.

PROGESTERONE

The reason women are given progesterone alongside oestrogen is to protect the uterine lining. But there isn't evidence at this stage that natural progesterone will provide long-term protection against breast cancer so we don't routinely give it to women who've had a hysterectomy. Progesterone doesn't protect against breast cancer, it just doesn't seem to increase the risk if natural progesterone is used within the first five years of HRT. Natural progesterone often has other benefits also. It can have a calming effect and help women sleep. It doesn't seem to work in every woman however. Some women seem to be more sensitive to progesterone. In those instances we ask them to insert them vaginally.

TESTOSTERONE

We don't currently have a testosterone preparation which is licensed for women in the UK, so we prescribe it 'off licence'. It doesn't mean it doesn't work if it hasn't been regulated but it can mean it's more difficult for women to obtain and there may be less scientific evidence for safety and effectiveness. A menopause specialist may readily prescribe testosterone, whereas a GP or gynaecologist not trained in hormones possibly won't, as they may not feel confident of what it does and what doses are needed. There is a testosterone brand licensed in Australia which unfortunately isn't licensed here yet; we hope to change that.

What many women don't realise is that testosterone is a female hormone and in fact they produce four times as much testosterone as oestrogen. As women age, the levels of testosterone in the body decline and below a certain level, some women start to get problems. They may notice loss of libido and arousal. There may also be a loss of energy and women often describe brain 'fog'. As soon as they start using testosterone, many regain their mental clarity and their zest for life which is vitally important.

WHAT'S THE DIFFERENCE BETWEEN BIO AND BODY IDENTICAL HRT?

The terms bioidentical and body identical both refer to hormones that are biochemically the same as the hormones made by your body, which are usually derived from soy and yams. They are terms that are both used to mean the same thing.

Regulated bioidentical hormone replacement therapy (rBHRT) refers to body identical hormones that are available on a standard, regulated prescription either on the NHS or privately. They include oestradiol and micronised progesterone and are often better tolerated and have fewer health risks (including breast cancer) when compared with their synthetic alternatives. Testosterone is also a bioidentical hormone that is available for prescription 'off license' which means it isn't licensed in the UK for female use, but GP and consultant menopause specialists will prescribe it if they're confident in doing so.

Compounded bioidentical hormone replacement therapy (cBHRT) is not conventionally regulated and not available on the NHS. Some clinics offer compounded bioidentical HRT as a 'custom-blended' treatment. They are marketed as precise duplicates of the hormones from your ovaries after blood test analysis. The hormone combination is then made up by a private pharmacy. However, unlike conventionally regulated biodentical HRT, compounded bioidentical HRT is not subject to the same rigorous testing for safety and effectiveness.

The blood tests and compounded hormones are also expensive – significantly more than the cost of a conventional prescription. More expensive does not necessarily mean better.

ARE ENOUGH GPs TRAINED IN THE MENOPAUSE?

No, I don't believe so; although more GPs are taking an active interest in menopause and are working towards British Menopause Society certification to enhance their knowledge within this area. I work in a busy hospital menopause service but the number of hospital clinics is limited. What we need within every general practice is at least one keen GP interested in women's health and menopause to manage most of the cases. The more difficult cases can be referred to hospital or menopause specialist clinics.

GPs are vital. I feel very strongly that menopause should be a key part of their training – both at undergraduate and graduate levels. I'd like to see more trainees routinely rotating through menopause clinics in our hospitals. The British Menopause Society and the Faculty of Sexual and Reproductive Healthcare have a menopause certification which can be taken at a basic or advanced level whereby you become a specialist within the area. The Royal College of Obstetricians and Gynaecologists (RCOG) have an Advanced Training Skills module in menopause so it is possible for gynaecologists to get training in this area.

I would like to see more emphasis on menopause in the core curriculum of all GPs. I work closely with GPs (my wife is a menopause specialist GP) and their work is very important. I'd also like more to train as menopause specialists so women can get the help they need more quickly."

—— **Mr Nick Panay** ——

As Mr Panay says, not enough GPs are trained in the specialist area of hormones and the menopause – yet – and if you're experiencing peri or menopausal symptoms, it can sometimes be difficult to get the help you need straight away. That's exactly my own experience. As I explained earlier, one GP I saw prescribed me antidepressants instead of recognising I was menopausal and therefore needed something more targeted.

So I was delighted when I came across the **My Menopause Centre** website while I was researching the whole topic of the menopause for this book.

It's an online service for women that offers free, evidence-based information and advice on all stages of the menopause transition, thirty-eight (yes, thirty-eight!) symptoms of the menopause and an algorithmically-driven questionnaire that results in a personalised menopause assessment.

It was launched in April 2021 by **Dr Clare Spencer**, a GP and menopause specialist from Leeds and **Helen Normoyle**, her long-term friend, a self-described well-being warrior. (My Menopause Centre also provides an online, private menopause clinic, run by doctors who specialise in the treatment of the menopause, led by Dr Spencer.)

As it's still a relatively new service, many women still won't have heard of it so I thought it was important to include here. First of all, meet Helen Normoyle who explains how and why My Menopause Centre came about:

"CLARE and I had been friends for several years before the idea for My Menopause Centre, having become friends outside of the school gates in 2012. Over the course of the last decade, Clare, a practicing GP, noticed a need for increased awareness and understanding of the menopause transition amongst her patients. As well as her own challenging menopause experience, she could see how their menopause symptoms were having a detrimental impact on all aspects of her patients' lives and made the decision to qualify as a registered menopause specialist.

When I became aware that I was going through the menopause, the symptoms I started to experience came as a complete surprise and I was consequently very unprepared for what was coming my way. One afternoon I found myself sitting on Clare's sofa asking lots of questions about the menopause, symptoms and treatment. I left our conversation feeling very reassured thanks to Clare's specialist advice but also wondered why it was so difficult to find easy-to-understand, evidence-based information and advice on what I was experiencing and the different treatment options. And so, the idea for My Menopause Centre was born.

My Menopause Centre is completely self-funded by myself and Clare. We're both incredibly driven by a purpose-led mission to reach everyone with free, impartial, evidence-based information and advice about the menopause. In order to do this, at its core, the service is completely advert-free. It is vitally important to us as the co-founders that our personal experiences and expertise contribute to a joint vision that is, at its heart, authentic and a driver for societal change. More widely, the centre offers private appointments with doctors who are menopause experts, as well as consultancy to businesses in the form of workshops and advice. It is this model that combines purpose, impartiality and accessibility to all, with a private clinic, that is at the heart of the business.

The Centre is an online clinic and website that has been created to empower women to take control of their menopause and thrive with evidence-based information and advice from menopause experts. Our research shows that knowledge is power; the more prepared a woman is for the menopause, the better her experience of it will be. While only one in four women say they feel/

felt prepared for the menopause, those who say they feel prepared are far more likely than other women to say that menopause can be a positive change in women's lives and less likely to say they feel/felt under pressure just to cope with the symptoms and less likely to say they feel/felt more isolated from others as a result of the menopause.

That's why at My Menopause Centre, we're determined to make the menopause **everyone's business**, and are passionate about empowering people across the UK – women of all ages, their partners and children, and men in general – with free and evidence-based support and tools. We understand the power of robust, quality information in giving women the freedom to make choices about their treatment.

By gathering information about the symptoms of the menopause experienced by women through our online questionnaire, we are also passionate about using Femtech (technology to support women's health) to bridge the health data gap that exists today to generate pioneering insights – including by age and ethnicity - that will enable us to truly tailor and develop our services and place the voices of all women at the centre of their delivery.

We need to get past this notion that the menopause only affects those experiencing it. It affects everyone, and its impact is far reaching from our homes to our workplaces. Society will continue to exacerbate the negative impact of the menopause on women until younger women and men of all ages join the conversation and educate themselves on what to expect and how to talk to a loved one experiencing it."

—— **Helen Normoyle** ——

Now here's Dr Clare Spencer who sees women dealing with menopausal symptoms in her Leeds GP practice and via The Menopause Centre:

IN YOUR EXPERIENCE, WHAT ARE THE MOST COMMON MENOPAUSAL SYMPTOMS?

"THE symptoms that women talk about most frequently in clinic - after hot flushes - are symptoms that relate to how their brain functions – so brain fog, poor concentration, memory loss and word finding difficulties. Women often tell me that they 'don't feel themselves'; that they feel more anxious about tasks they would ordinarily deal with, or they are suffering out of the blue low mood for no reason. For some women, these symptoms can slowly creep up on them over the course of the perimenopause.

I also hear frequently about vaginal symptoms - vaginal dryness, irritation and pain during sex. These symptoms are frequently not volunteered until I ask specifically about them, as many women are too embarrassed to discuss them.

ARE THERE REASONS WHY HRT WOULD NOT BE RECOMMENDED OR POSSIBLE TO PRESCRIBE FOR SOME WOMEN?

For the vast majority of women, the benefits of HRT outweigh the risks and there are very few contraindications to HRT. There are a minority of women for whom HRT may be unsuitable. Every single woman should be treated as an individual and the risks and benefits of taking HRT should be weighed up both for and with them. Where HRT is likely to be more risky, or where the evidence is uncertain, I would strongly recommend a discussion with a menopause specialist.

Some forms of HRT are safer than others. For example, oestrogen taken in tablet form increases the risk of blood clots and stroke, whereas oestrogen taken through the skin (transdermally) does not. Some women are at greater risk of blood clots and stroke - this may be because of a medical condition or previous blood clots, or they may be obese, smoke or suffer from migraines. For these women it's safer to use transdermal oestrogen rather than tablet form.

If women suffer from migraine with aura, the risk of stroke can be increased. Women can take HRT, but it should be through the skin rather than tablet form.

IF HRT IS NOT SUITABLE, WHAT OTHER WAYS CAN A WOMAN NAVIGATE THE MENOPAUSE?

There are various options to help women navigate the menopause other than HRT:

Lifestyle changes: It will not surprise you to know that there is evidence that tackling diet and exercise can help in the management of menopause symptoms. Exercise helps with weight management and helps manage the risk of cardiovascular disease. Weight-bearing exercise is great for helping to prevent osteoporosis – and these are both long-term health consequences of the menopause.

Avoiding rich food, spicy food, alcohol and caffeine can be helpful in preventing hot flushes. There is evidence that a Mediterranean style diet can help keep the risk of heart disease down.

Cutting down on alcohol consumption - many women choose alcohol to self-medicate to help them sleep and take the edge off anxiety and stress. Alcohol is a depressant, so can make mood symptoms worse, and interferes with sleep also.

MEDICATION THAT IS NOT HRT

There are some available. However these will only address symptoms and won't have the same long-term health benefits HRT has in reducing the risk of cardiovascular disease and osteoporosis:

Clonidine is a tablet that is used for blood pressure, and this has also been shown to be helpful in the management of hot flushes.

Antidepressants have a role to play in managing menopause symptoms, particularly for women who have been advised not to take HRT, or do not wish to take HRT. They can be helpful in managing mood and they can help manage hot flushes and night sweats. Women taking Tamoxifen for breast cancer should be aware that some (but not all) antidepressants can make the drug less effective.

Pregabalin and gabapentin are medications that are used more commonly for pain, anxiety, prevention of migraine, depression, anxiety and epilepsy. They can also be helpful in managing hot flushes and helping sleep (off license use).

Duloxetine and oxybutynin have also been used for the management of hot flushes.

HERBAL ALTERNATIVES AND SUPPLEMENTS

There are various herbal remedies on the market. Many women turn to herbal remedies before seeing a doctor for advice. If you are investigating herbal solutions, always look for the THR mark on the box:

The Traditional Herbal Registration certification means the product has been registered by the Medicines and Healthcare products Regulatory Agency under the UK Traditional Herbal Registration Scheme.

When thinking about herbal remedies, you should consider the fact that the strength and safety are not fully known, that multiple preparation types exist and we don't know which is the safest or best. And it's important to also know that herbal medicines can interfere with medicines that are prescribed by doctors.

Many women choose to try St John's Wort. It was mentioned in the National Institute of Excellence (NICE) Menopause guidance NG23. It may be beneficial in treating anxiety and depression, but it is important to bear in mind that St John's Wort can make certain medicines less effective. It should not be taken with antidepressants, digoxin, warfarin, anti-asthma drugs, oral contraceptives, migraine drugs, cancer drugs and HIV drugs. This list isn't exhaustive – please check with a doctor if you are thinking about taking St John's Wort.

Women in the perimenopause and menopause are at greater risk of osteoporosis – thinning of the bones – and fractures. Vitamin D and calcium are important in providing the body with essential bone building blocks. Taking a vitamin D supplement through the winter months is therefore recommended for everyone and is all the more important if you are transitioning through the menopause and beyond.

HOW ARE DOCTORS LINKED TO THE CENTRE RECRUITED?

The sad truth is that there are not as many trained menopause doctors in the UK as we need. For that reason, we have been able to use our connections and word of mouth to recruit the very best doctors who are not only highly qualified but share our goals of listening to their patients, understanding their needs and goals, and empowering them with the information and advice to make the choices that are best for them."

—— **Dr Clare Spencer** ——

"WE passionately believe that as a society, we need to reframe the menopause and reframe what it means to be a middle-aged woman. Over the last century the average life expectancy for a woman has increased considerably – in 1921 life expectancy at birth for a woman was fifty-nine and she went through the menopause at fifty-seven.

One hundred years later, the average woman in her fifties can expect to live until eighty-seven and she'll go through the menopause at fifty-one. What this means is that ever more of a woman's life will be lived postmenopausal (thirty-six years, or forty per cent of the life of today's average fifty-something woman). Who wants to be written off when the second half of life is still ahead? Our research has shown that women who were prepared for the menopause had better outcomes and were more likely to agree that menopause can be a positive change.

This reluctance to discuss and acknowledge the menopause (at home as well as at work) is also wrapped up in ageism. We live in an ageist society that venerates youth so by sharing her menopausal status, a woman is linking herself to an important marker in the ageing process – that she is nearing the end of her fertility, and we wonder if there is something conscious or subconscious coming into play at this point about a woman's value in society when she can no longer bear children.

As a consequence, when middle-aged/menopausal women are represented, it is too often in an ageist and stereotypical way, with their symptoms such as hot flushes or mood changes, the butt of jokes or discussed in a sexist and derogatory way.

A survey by UK by UM in 2018 found older women feel stereotyped in advertising with sixty-one per cent of menopausal women agreeing society expects them to vanish from public life as they get older. And a report by L'Oréal found despite forty per cent of women being over fifty (the fastest growing demographic), over fifties represent only fifteen per cent of the women we see in the media. Is it any wonder that so many women are reluctant to discuss what they are going through, or ask for the help and support they need whether at home or at work?"

—— **Dr Clare Spencer and Helen Normoyle** ——

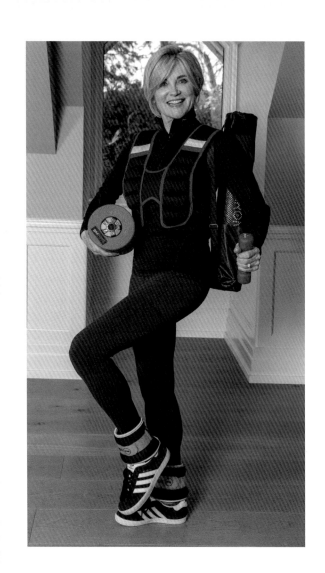

CHAPTER II

—— *Fitness and Exercise* ——

IT'S so important to move - and keep moving. Your fitness choices can take any guise you like to suit your age, stamina and ability – just as long as you move every day! I studied ballet until the age of nineteen and although I've done little since, it has left me with an understanding of what the body is capable of and what I expect to be able to do. For me it's unimaginable not to have a full range of movement and it's fear and a sense of gratitude that's kept me moving on a daily basis.

If I had to pick an area which I give the most attention to it's core strength. I believe it's an area you should work on as everything feeds into it; together with your mind, it's your power.

I competed in the Channel 4 show *SAS Who Dares Wins* presented by Ant Middleton (yes, I was nicknamed Grandma) and there was one exercise where I knew if I engaged my core together with my mind, I'd got this; leave either of them on the beach and I was going to hurt like hell. A helicopter hovers many meters over a cold Scottish sea, there is no door and you are standing on the foot trim facing into the helicopter looking at Ant. You place your arms across your chest and he pushes you backwards so you lose your balance. If you can hold your nerve and your stomach muscles you will invert by the sheer weight of your head and hit the sea clean head-first, straight as an arrow.

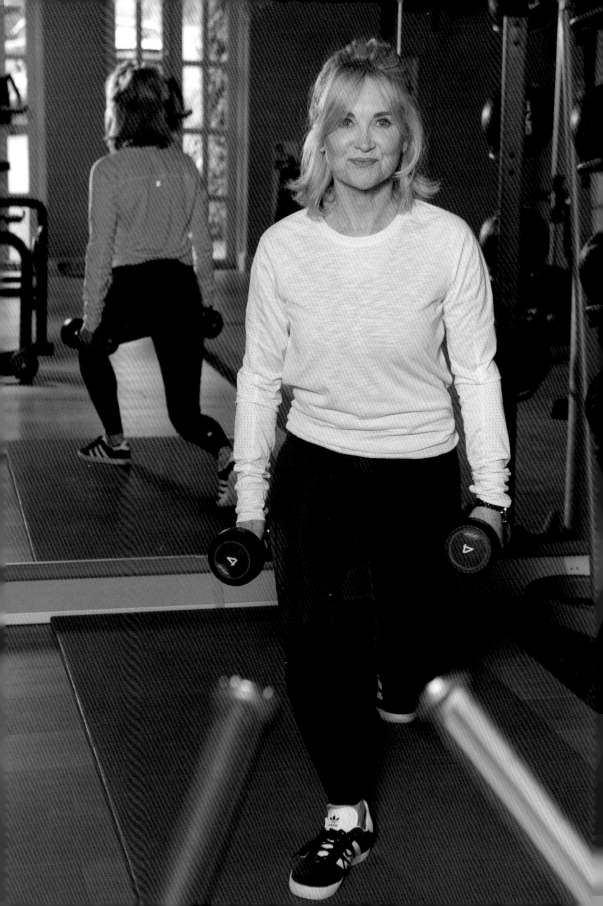

When I eventually got to shore (I'm a rubbish swimmer) Olli Ollerton, the former SAS soldier on the programme, looked at me and said, 'Text book'. That's all I needed, my time was up, I'd done it for all us 'Grandmas'.

I'm not a trained fitness expert so I can't tell you what you should and shouldn't do. I can only tell you what I do and what I have found works for me.

I try and do something active every day. I don't have a set routine and I don't limit myself to any one exercise. I'm happy to try anything and everything within reason. The lockdowns taught us that we don't need to go to the gym if we choose not to; we can move either at home or outside in the fresh air with or without equipment. I'm not a great runner in fact I don't enjoy it but I do feel better once I've made myself get out there. I do no more than just twenty minutes out, twenty minutes back and totally applaud people who do more. If you've not done any running before, just start off walking and gradually pick up the pace. It's not about doing a marathon or running for hours; it's more about keeping our bodies active and raising the heart rate.

The scientist Dr Norman Lazarus (I can't stop reading his book, *The Lazarus Strategy*) stresses the importance of moving, no matter what it is. He says whether you choose ballroom dancing or running, exercise should be enjoyable and should raise your heart rate to at least sixty per cent of its maximum. That's what I aim for.

As an ageing woman I've learnt the importance of weights to avoid osteoporosis. A few years ago, I was diagnosed with osteopenia which is the warning sign that if you don't make a few adjustments you could end up with osteoporosis. Taking this on board, I swapped my tablet HRT to Body Identical, took a high value Vitamin D supplement morning and night , increased my resistance work, cut down on sugar and on my last test I had successfully arrested the situation.

The last thing we want is osteoporosis which can lead to bones fracturing more easily which means pain, six weeks recovery (minimum), possibly being unable to work, travel and enjoy daily life.

I sometimes use a gym and perform a few weight-bearing exercises on the various machines. More often I use free weights at home or in my latest multi-tasking brainwave to make Soho's dog walks productive for us both I've invested in a 6kg weight vest and 2kg ankle weights, so while Soho is sniffing his hundredth blade of grass, I can get on with a few squats and leg raises. Adding weights to yourself or holding weights forces your muscles to work harder which builds them up giving you a better shape. Weight-bearing burns calories and puts stress on the bones which encourages bone-forming cells to raise their game.

— *A* —

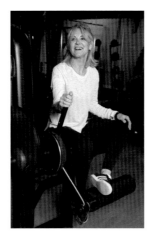
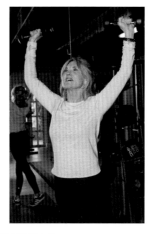

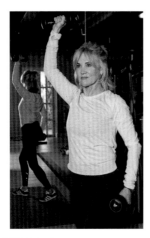
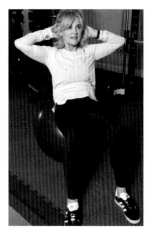

ENJOYING MY GYM SESSION!

Fitness expert and author **Paula Kerr**, created the hugely successful fitness brand Fitter Stronger in her forties, proving it's never too late to get fit! Here she offers her tips on exercise as we get older:

"AS we age, we need to work on three exercise areas:

- Improving stamina
- Increasing muscle density
- Developing core strength

Stamina, muscle density and core strength are needed for the activities we do every day. They provide our functional fitness, flexibility and confidence in our bodies, as we grow older. We want to be able to lift our shopping out of a car without damaging our back, to climb steps without becoming breathless or unsteady, to remove a heavy object from a high shelf or walk on sand, knowing our bodies will serve us well.

After age thirty-five, our metabolism slows down, reducing our stamina and energy levels, causing weight gain. At this time, our muscle and bone density begins to lessen. The good news is that all of these things can be counteracted with a balanced diet and regular exercise.

If you are new to exercise, are recovering from illness or injury or have had a long pause since your last exercise session, always consult a doctor before you begin. Always mobilise your muscles before you begin to exercise and stretch them afterwards, to release tension and prevent muscle soreness.

Start by committing to thirty minutes of movement, three times a week. Choose an exercise that you like, that will test your muscles and increase your heart rate and stick with it. Ideally, choose a mix of exercise types, to prevent boredom.

Exercise doesn't have to be expensive or complicated. It can be as simple as pulling on a pair of trainers and going for a half-hour walk. Use your walk to improve stamina, by walking to the next tree but speed walking, jogging or sprinting to the one after. Continue for five minutes and walk for the remaining twenty-five minutes. Each time you repeat this, add a minute to your jogging sections, until you can comfortably continue for twenty minutes and the walking breaks are shorter. Build muscle density further by utilising park benches for tricep dips or stopping every five minutes for twenty squats or jumping squats or sit-ups.

Try to get into nature as often as possible, which benefits our mental health, by releasing endorphins that will calm the stress hormone, cortisol.

JUST DO IT

Avoid making excuses! If you have upper body issues, stay with leg exercises. If you have lower body issues, build upper body and core strength while seated or laying down, within your capability. If you can't run, jog or walk. Be consistent and patient. Give yourself twelve weeks for significant results. Don't do a ten-minute run once a fortnight and wonder why you aren't ready for your first marathon yet.

Choose exercise that reflects your energy level, ability and agility. If you are short on time or energy, choose a shorter workout. If you are feeling strong and energised, choose a more challenging workout and move for a longer time.

If you prefer to exercise at home, consider investing in a few versatile, inexpensive items, which might include dumbbells (hand weights), a mat and a skipping rope, all of which are easily available. If you don't have them, improvise with household items that you can safely utilise. If you don't have hand weights, try water bottles filled with water or sand, according to your required resistance.

YOUR STRENGTH IS YOUR CORE

Include some core strength exercises every week. The stronger your core muscles become, the more effective your other exercises will be. Your running style will improve as you hold your posture better and you will be able to lift heavier weights, as your core supports your lumbar spine. Our core muscles support our lower back. When they are weak, we are more susceptible to lower back pain.
I feel energised when I play music during exercise, whether this is a work-out or a run. Put a playlist together that inspires and invigorates you.

If you have no medical impairment and have exercised before, train for up to an hour each time, giving each session everything you've got. Make the most of the time you have allocated to improve your strength, endurance, stamina and flexibility. Use weights that will challenge you, but can be lifted safely. Whatever your level, always go for good form over high reps. Take as many breaks as you need and move at your own pace.

Always warm up before every exercise session and stretch your muscles after your workout.

Do each of these actions for at least fifteen seconds. Start with a jog on the spot, gradually increasing speed. Bring your knees up in front of you. Return to a jog on the spot. Kick your heels up behind you. Return to a jog on the spot. Rotate your hips in big circles. After five rotations, change direction and repeat. Roll your shoulders. Rotate your arms, gradually lifting your arms higher, until your elbows sweep past your ears. Repeat, taking your arms in the opposite direction. Turn your head so that you can see your right shoulder. Bring your head back to a neutral position. Then, turn your head so that you can see your left shoulder. Return your head to a neutral position. Look up to the ceiling, then down to the floor. Return your head to a neutral position. Take your right ear towards your right shoulder, then your left ear towards your left shoulder. Return your head to a neutral position. If the warm up presents no pain, continue with your exercise.

If you have tight muscles, visit a physio or sports massage therapist to help these ease. Remember to take rest days. A regular pattern of three days of exercise followed by one day of rest works well and allows the muscles to relax and repair.

KEEP IT REGULAR

Regular exercise reduces blood pressure and creates an anti-inflammatory reaction in the body, reducing pain caused by osteo or rheumatoid arthritis. If you have muscular skeletal pain and you don't exercise, the muscles around your joints become weaker. The joints are then unsupported by strong muscle. If there is joint destruction, you need good muscle strength to support those joints. In many cases, you can delay or avoid surgery by increasing muscle density.

As well as physical improvement, exercise is a great stress buster, which is hugely useful to those coping with poor mental health or impacted by illness or injury. You can't out train a bad diet. No amount of exercise will make you fit and strong if you have bad nutrition. For maximum benefit, eat a little protein and fruit or vegetables with every meal. Protein rich food, such as lean poultry and eggs, will aid your body in repairing from daily exertion and help to satiate appetite. A colourful variety of fruit and vegetables will provide the majority of vitamins and minerals required for organ function and a supported immune system."

—— **Paula Kerr** ——

YOGA

As I say, when it comes to exercise, a bit of everything works for me. I enjoy doing weights, a bit of running, walking and Pilates. Friends of mine extol the benefits of yoga which is said to be especially good for women who may never have exercised or got out of the habit of exercising.

Whatever your body type, whatever your fitness level, I guarantee there is a yoga class out there for you. It depends on what you're looking for. As we get older, flexibility gets more and more important after years of sitting at a desk perhaps or running around less than we used to. Personally, that's what I want to achieve when I do exercise, that and maintaining my all-round strength.

There are so many different types of yoga - Iyengar yoga, Ashtanga, Vinyasa, Bikram and Yin to name just a few - and if you're a newbie, don't let this put you off. Some classes move faster than others, some are gentle and meditative but at the end of every yoga class experts say you should feel so much better, physically and mentally.

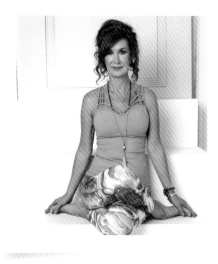

REGINA KERSCHBAUMER

Surrey-based **Regina Kerschbaumer**, the creator and founder of Yoga Orchid and Yoga Orchid Yinstitute, practices and teaches Yin yoga which is a more passive form of yoga and consists of longer-held floor poses which tend to work the lower part of the body including the lower spine. Regi is in her fifties (although you'd never know it to look at her!) and strongly believes everyone can benefit from practicing yoga, no matter what age.

"PEOPLE often say, 'I can't do yoga, I'm not flexible enough,' or 'I'm overweight. Once I lose weight I will take up yoga.' But yoga will help with all of that. You're not too dirty to take a bath or you're not too hungry to eat! If you feel inflexible, yoga can help you regain your flexibility. If you're struggling with weight issues, yoga can help you lose weight. You're never too old to start with some gentle yoga and then gradually build up your fitness level and ability.

Yoga is a science of body, mind and soul; it's not just a physical exercise, there's much more to it than that.

Yoga specifically targets the spine. When we move the spine in its full functional range of motion – forwards, backwards, twisting, lateral stretching – we are not only keeping our spine healthy but I believe we're keeping our brain healthy. The brain and spinal cord is one organ - they are connected and make up the central nervous system. If you have a healthy spine you have a healthy body and if you have a flexible back you will have a flexible mind. Our bodies are vehicles of expression and if you're rigid and inflexible, your mind can become like that also.

Yoga is a progressive practice. We start gradually doing gentle movements like 'downward dog' which will strengthen your muscles and eventually you're strong enough to go on to handstands. Last week I had a sixty-nine year-old man in my class going up on a handstand! It's so uplifting for the yogis to be able to do things with their bodies that they never thought would be possible. You have to keep moving and use your body in every possible way you can to stay young and healthy!

When we go back to the floor and do slow, long, holds, we do Yin yoga. We hold the postures in a relaxed way for two to five minutes to stretch the joints, which helps us to regain our flexibility.

There are over two thousand yoga poses. If a teacher is experienced enough, they will be able to adjust a class to suit all levels and abilities. If you can't do a pose because of your physical limitations or a health condition then there will always be an alternative posture to do which will give you the same benefit. Remember you cannot do it wrong. Yoga is not about being good at it; it is about the physical and mental benefits you will gain from it.

Yoga is a wonderful complement and sports enhancer to other forms of exercise like running, golf, tennis or swimming.

Yoga teaches us to breathe properly - nostril breathing, deep into the belly - which helps us to tap into the parasympathetic nervous system and calms us down. The breath is the anchor of all styles of yoga. The breath is life, it gives us energy, vitality and keeps us alive. Breath awareness brings us into the present moment and teaches us mindfulness.

I started yoga at thirty-one and never looked back. I was a young mum at the time with two toddlers. I just wanted something for myself and found a yoga class - or shall I say yoga found me. I can do more things with my body now than when I was thirty and I feel just as healthy as when I was sixteen. Yoga wasn't very widespread at the time and I think my friends thought I'd joined some sort of cult! Fortunately, there's been a big shift since and the world has woken up to yoga, mindfulness and meditation.

Yoga brings a balance back into the body, it helps you to regain your joint flexibility, muscular strength, organ health and it improves your balance. It improves your posture and can take years off your biological age! Most of all it quiets the mind and nourishes the soul. Yoga satisfies many different needs; it's a way of life."

—— **Regina Kerschbaumer** ——

ALEXANDER TECHNIQUE

> You are as old as your spine
>
> Chinese proverb

I am fascinated by watching people doing everyday things – standing, sitting, walking and so on – and seeing how they do it. I do believe if you can understand how humans move, how we moved when we were kids, you will understand how vital it is to move properly as adults. Years ago I learned the Alexander Technique, and I incorporate the movements I was taught, into my everyday life and activities. It's about standing tall, holding in your core, pushing back your shoulders and using your body how it was designed to be used. It might sound complicated but it really isn't. In my opinion, all you really need to keep in mind is how vital it is to keep your body moving.

I recently reengaged with the Alexander Technique when I visited the Constructive Teaching Centre in London and watched teachers being trained so they can help others. It reminded me how useful the technique is in my everyday life so I asked **Duncan Knowles**, the Centre's Assistant to the Director of Training, to try and explain a bit more about the AT:

WHAT IS THE ALEXANDER TECHNIQUE?

"THE Alexander Technique teaches people to greatly improve their well-being in daily life, and in activities of all kinds. It is often described in terms related to movement and posture, and while it does encompass these elements, its scope is much broader – emphasising what F. Matthias Alexander (1867–1955), its progenitor, described as 'the use of the self'.

Alexander, an actor, experienced vocal and breathing difficulties that threatened his career. Conventional cures proved unsuccessful, so he took to painstaking self-observation. He determined that he was unconsciously disrupting the carriage and balance of his head while speaking, by tightening and stiffening unnecessarily and interfering with the use of his head, neck and back. Debilitating neuromuscular reactions resulted, causing the imbalance between these parts to radiate throughout his body and leading to a systemic lowering of his general functioning and well-being. He soon realised that these harmful reactions were not just restricted to speaking, but occurred in all acts of living.

HEALTH BENEFITS

Alexander's insight was to recognise that his use directly affected his functioning. But when he tried to stop the misuse of his head, neck and back, he found that his conscious ability to change his reactions was hindered by ingrained unconscious habits. He evolved his technique further, regaining full control over his use, including his voice and breathing.

Thus, how we organise ourselves as we go about our daily activities will have direct consequences for our well-being: if we can stop interfering with our general functioning – respiration, circulation, digestion, neuromuscular and skeletal systems, etc. – then we can invite greater health, poise and vitality in our lives.

The health benefits are wide-ranging. Good use of our selves promotes appropriate functioning, while poorer use can lead to gradual deterioration.

Anyone can benefit from the Technique, no matter how old or young. (I recently had an eighty-year-old pupil who found it challenging to walk; her lessons left her much more mobile, and a lot happier.)

HOW IS IT DIFFERENT FROM EXERCISE?

'The Alexander Technique is a method of self-help,' explained one of the Technique's greatest exponents, Walter Carrington. '... Unlike most systems that advise people what to do and how to do it, it teaches us what not to do and how to prevent it.' As Alexander was known to say: 'If you can stop doing the wrong thing, the right thing will do itself.'

There are no exercises in the Alexander Technique. Because it is designed to stop unhelpful reactions that have negative consequences for the whole postural mechanism, it's actually a precursor to exercise – or to any activity.

In practical terms, we guide people to re-establish helpful patterns of use. With the improved functioning that follows, they can better meet their potential in all areas of their lives. This approach is very rewarding for people involved in exercise, sports, any activities that require a high degree of skill, mobility and balance, where marginal gains can be important.

HAVING LESSONS

During a lesson, the teacher works with the pupil to discern the latter's neuromuscular responses as they carry out simple movements and activities such as standing and sitting in a chair. The teacher guides the pupil to change unhelpful patterns and reactions that interfere with their general well-being and functioning, as Alexander himself did. Chair work is supplemented by table work, during which the pupil lies semi-supine on a table: with the aid of gravity, the body can return to a healthier, more natural alignment.

As lessons progress, we look at other activities such as walking, lifting, sitting at a desk and so on – at any activity, in fact, that is of interest to the pupil.

Thirty lessons over three to six months makes for a very good foundation in the Technique. This is roughly the model I like follow. It isn't always feasible for people with busy schedules, and many pupils have derived great benefit from different, less concentrated approaches.

It's easy to find an Alexander Technique teacher online, and we offer private lessons at the Constructive Teaching Centre."

—— **Duncan Knowles** ——

While at the Constructive Teaching Centre, I spoke to some Alexander Technique teachers and trainees. What they all had in common was the belief that the Technique has helped them in their daily lives, often alieviating physical pain or stress.

Forty-five year-old Jen Elkeles explains here what drew her to the AT and why she's now training to become a teacher.

"I was drawn to the Alexander technique because of pain. I had suffered with sciatica (where the sciatic nerve which runs from the lower back to your feet is compressed) for several years. This started in my late thirties/early forties (sciatica often affects people in their forties and fifties). Once or twice a year I'd have a very painful episode lasting a couple of months or so. I took eight to ten painkillers a day and I had to lie down - a lot. I tried several things including osteopathy, Pilates and physio. I didn't find anything particularly helpful and actually tensing and bracing my abdominal muscles resulted in my lower back feeling even tighter and more uncomfortable.

When I was forty-four, what I thought was an unwelcome flare up, turned into something quite different. The pain was on a scale I hadn't experienced before and it became intolerable. I couldn't stand for more than about thirty seconds and I was pretty much immobile. After about four weeks I resorted to surgery which established that a piece of cartilage had come off one of the discs on my spine and had got embedded in the sciatic nerve. The whole experience, particularly the pain and lack of mobility, had left me feeling old beyond my years and I knew something had to change.

I was regaling my woes to a friend some weeks after my surgery who mentioned the Alexander Technique. I decided to book a lesson.

At the time of my first lesson I was out of pain. However, my back still felt very weak, rigid and stiff. My teacher (Susanna Scouller) worked on me with me lying on a table and also moving from sitting and standing in a chair. When sitting, Susanna guided me into an improved state of overall balance and co-ordination of my head, neck and back. I was struck by how unfamiliar sitting in this way felt and I was absolutely convinced that I was sitting at a forty-five degree angle forwards, practically doing a nose dive. Susanna took a photo and I was absolutely upright! I went for a walk the day after my first lesson and the feeling was quite extraordinary. I felt weightless, like I was walking on springs. I felt so light on my feet and in my legs I felt I could take off.

For the first time I feel like I have some control over my back. As I am learning to be aware of and inhibit harmful movement patterns and postural habits my muscular system is re-learning its sense of natural co-ordination so that the underworking muscles start working and the overworked ones release tension and do less. This benefits not just my back but my muscular skeletal system overall.

I started the teaching course at the Constructive Teaching Centre to learn how to keep myself out of pain and to gain a deeper understanding of how and why the technique works. I am absolutely loving it and would derive huge satisfaction from being able to pass onto others the benefits I have experienced, and to prevent and manage injury and pain.

As we restore our body's natural instinct for poise and muscle co-ordination it functions better as a whole - physically and mentally. The technique doesn't only help relieve back, neck and joint pain and muscle tension and stiffness; there are so many other benefits such as improving breathing, circulation, vocal problems, ease and freedom of movement and balance and stability. It also helps you to think more clearly and feel younger, lighter, taller, calmer and more confident. What's not to like!"

—— **Jen Elkeles** ——

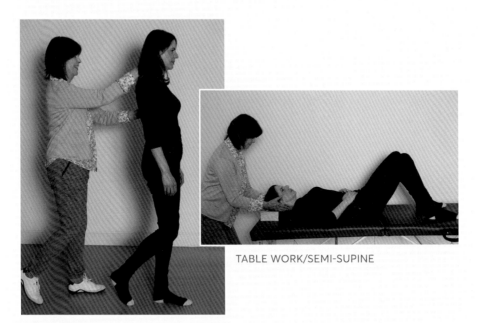

TABLE WORK/SEMI-SUPINE

WALKING

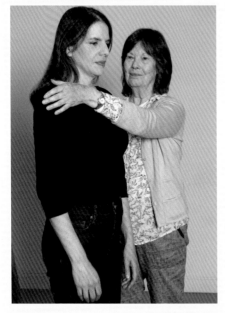

STANDING

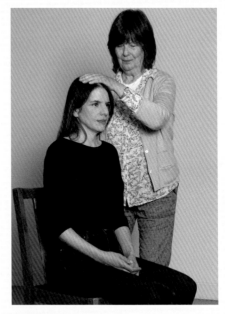

CHAIR WORK

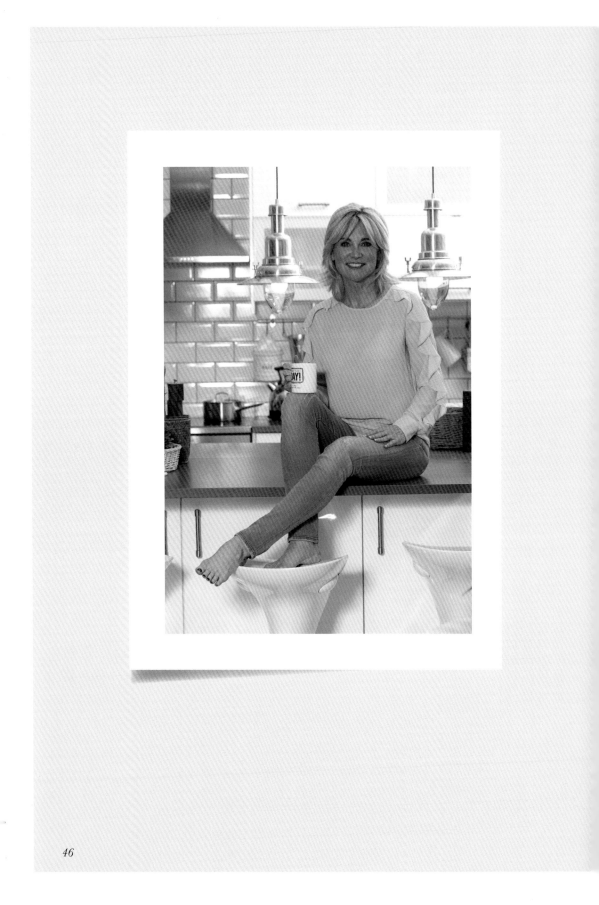

CHAPTER III

— Nutrition —

I LEAD a varied lifestyle. I don't do the same thing each day which means I don't have set meal times although I 'try' not to eat too late. But when I go to bed I take a collagen drink with me and I have found this has helped with joint and muscle aches and pains.

If I examine my changing eating patterns, one thing that I have realised is a constant is that the foods I consume are largely whole. I've eliminated from my diet most processed foods and I usually know the source of whatever it is I've eaten. Even if it's granola for instance, if I haven't made it myself, I research where it comes from and will pick a brand that is full of whole goodness. I like yogurt and make sure it's organic. I do have butter and know it's not full of additives and I prefer whole fruits to fruit juices.

On four days a week I don't really eat until after noon. This isn't for weight-loss reasons and not for everyone. I personally just prefer to eat this way. Holidays of course are different. There's nothing quite like a lovely hotel breakfast which someone has prepared for you with no washing up afterwards!

When I wake up, on an empty stomach I have a prebiotic powder mixed into a probiotic kefir. It doesn't taste great but I'll gulp it back and feel my gut is loving me for it.

Somewhere between 12 and 1pm, I will have something to eat. It will almost certainly involve an avocado, egg or tuna. I've definitely got Mediterranean tastes. If I had to pick one diet, it would be that. I eat olives like sweets. Again, if I'm meeting someone for lunch, this could change but my habit of knowing what I'm eating and keeping it as fresh and natural as possible, remains. Good quality coffee will most likely make an appearance and possibly a biscuit but only the one; no need for the whole packet!

I make sure I have carrots, peppers and humus in the fridge if I get a snack attack. I also have a nut jar everywhere I go with a nice collection of Brazil or walnuts.

As far as my evening meal is concerned, again I go back to tuna and vegetables, spiced up with herbs or garlic, never boring. Occasionally I will have a steak. I love potatoes and pasta but wouldn't have them too often. When I do, I enjoy them. My partner Mark is half Italian and grew up in a family in the sixties and seventies who enjoyed good food while we were still slopping out Coronation chicken! He loves nothing more than a bowl of pasta so if he says he wants it for dinner, I will enjoy it with him, just not every night.

If I'm out at a restaurant, I'll treat myself to a pudding but certainly not every time. I used to when I was younger; I was like a dustbin and ate whenever and whatever I wanted. Now I know I will put on weight so puddings have a warning sign over them. Of course I enjoy a glass of wine. Mainly I will have one large glass of red wine. It's sociable and red wines are better for you than white and contain antioxidants. Similarly, I adore chocolate but tend to stick to a couple of squares of dark chocolate only.

I'm not saying I don't enjoy beans on toast or fish and chips or even fish finger sandwiches but these are not foods I have every day. It's about taking control of your own body and doing what's right for you. If you want to stay slim as you age which I do, then I know I can't over indulge but nor do want a boring life and to deny myself life's pleasures. I feel I have found the right balance for my body.

— *A* —

Lorraine Nicolle is a Nutritionist and Nutritional Therapist and there's nothing she doesn't know about how to eat well! Here's what she has to say about my diet:

"WHAT a great start! Anthea is eating mainly natural whole foods and is having processed foods and added sugars only very occasionally. That is something that everybody can do and is probably the strongest nutritional game-changer if we are looking for good health as we age. Organic yoghurt can be a good source of protein and live bacteria for the gut, and butter can also be beneficial because it is one of the few dietary sources of pre-formed vitamin A and butyric acid, both of which are important in keeping the gastrointestinal lining strong.

And whole fruit is so much better than fruit juices because it contains all the natural fibre, so the sugar in the fruit is less disruptive to our metabolism. Fasting during the morning has become quite popular and for good reason because a lengthy overnight fast has been shown to contribute to weight loss and to help keep blood fats and inflammatory chemicals at lower levels. If Anthea would like to truly benefit from this she could delay her nutritional drink until after she has fasted overnight for between fourteen and sixteen hours.

The collagen supplemental protein, prebiotic and the kefir drink that Anthea is taking are all useful as we go through midlife and beyond. There are ways of getting these nutrients through food, such as eating an abundance of different plant fibres throughout the day, together with high-quality protein. And perhaps some bone broth for the collagen. But doing it through powders should also be beneficial, as long as she is prepared to put up with the taste and she feels well on it.

The lunch choices are beneficial, especially as Anthea wisely chooses high-quality protein. Eggs are true superfoods because the protein they contain is very easy to digest, absorb and use by the human body. And they're also packed full of healthy fats and molecules called phospholipids that are crucial for the membranes of all our cells and for helping the brain to work properly. If there's one thing that Anthea could do to improve her lunch it would be to increase the variety of vegetables in the salads so that she is going for as many different colours as possible. Each colour represents a different type of phytochemical, all of which have different powerful healthy ageing effects and are potently anti-inflammatory. And walnuts are one of the healthiest types of nut to eat because they are packed full of fibre and polyphenols that support cardiovascular health, not to mention having some essential omegas.

Anthea looks as if she plans ahead because she always has her fridge stocked with some veggies for snacks. That's a really good idea because having stuff on hand makes it less tempting to go for something we shouldn't.

She also includes some oily fish in her diet and that is crucial for the anti-inflammatory fats EPA and DHA. They help improve cardiovascular health, inflammation and they support mood, clear-thinking and memory as we age.

It's clear that Anthea listens to her body and she's aware that concentrated starches like potatoes and pasta, and too much sugar, have detrimental effects on her metabolism and so she's got used to avoiding these unless she's having a treat. And having treats is important, as Anthea says herself. It sounds as if she has a balanced approach to eating and that having a little of what she fancies now and then makes it easier for her to stick to the good stuff for the majority of the time. A lot of people find it helpful to think of the eighty:twenty rule, which means that for twenty per cent of the time you can have whatever you want.

If there is anything to improve, I would suggest that Anthea sets some regular times for eating, as she has said herself that she doesn't tend to have set meal times. Everything in the body works on the twenty-four-hour clock. This means that our biochemistry is healthier and happier when we have regular routines, and this includes eating at around the same time every day (and not at night)."

Lorraine has been helping people to age well for nearly twenty years using nutritional and lifestyle medicine to help her clients reach their full health potential. Here she answers the questions we all have as we strive for good health as we grow older:

DO OUR NUTRIONAL NEEDS CHANGE AS WE AGE?

"Indeed they do, not least because of changing hormones, but also because of the accumulated 'allostatic load' over the years. Put simply, our state of health is influenced by everything that has happened throughout our life. Each experience has had an impact on the way our genes and cells function, meaning that the older we get, the more our body and brain have been affected by accumulated stressors.

The impact of this is that as we get into middle age and beyond we see that certain body systems may start to feel overburdened, and may need extra support nutritionally. We may experience this in flagging energy levels, lower alcohol tolerance (more hangovers!), feeling less refreshed after sleep, gaining weight more easily, general aches and pains, forgetfulness, feeling more apathetic and losing our joie de vivre. We may also find it harder to control our blood sugar levels, and this can have a huge impact on our ability to handle stress and function well day-to-day.

What's even more concerning to many is that gradually flagging body systems drive an increase in inflammation as we age. This may start out insidiously, but if not kept in check, this inflammation triggers degenerative diseases like arthritis, osteoporosis, cardiovascular disease, diabetes, dementia and cancer. This concept is commonly referred to as inflammaging.

Everyone's nutritional needs will be different, but in broad terms, as women get into mid-life, we tend to do better when we:

- **Increase protein** to support the muscle and bone mass that we're losing every year. Good sources of protein are fish (sustainably caught), and organic and outdoor reared meat, poultry and eggs. Organic dairy is also a healthy protein source for those of us lucky enough to be able to tolerate it. Vegans can get high quality protein by eating tofu and tempeh, and by combining whole grains with nuts and seeds, or with beans and pulses.

- **Reduce sugars and starches** in order to support healthy blood glucose and insulin levels and maintain a healthy weight. Every time you need sugar or starch you trigger a spike in insulin. Insulin is a fat storage hormone so this will hamper efforts to lose weight as we get older. Sugars are found in anything that has added sugars, as well as too much fruit (two to three pieces a day is enough), fruit juices and white grains or anything made from white flour.

 - **Get plenty of omega 3 fats** because these are anti-inflammatory. The most anti-inflammatory type of omega 3s are found in oily fish. Other types of omega 3s are found in flaxseeds and chia seeds. Some omega 6 fats are also important for hormonal and skin health in particular, and these can be found in nuts and seeds. And, in addition, unfiltered olive oil is a hugely helpful part of the everyday diet, because it supports cardiovascular health and is also loaded with polyphenols that are antioxidant and anti-inflammatory.

- **Eat eight to ten portions of vegetables a day.** One portion is approximately 80g and many people find it helpful to weigh their portions for the first two or three days until they get used to knowing what 80g of a vegetable looks like. Ten portions might sound like a lot but this can be easily done if you have four at lunch, four at dinner and then a couple as snacks.

- **Get plenty of prebiotic foods** that act as antioxidants and anti-inflammatories in the body, as well as feeding the microbes in the gut that are so crucial in controlling inflammation and general health. Here, we're talking about anything that includes fibre and variety is the best way to go. So get plenty of nuts, seeds, beans and pulses, vegetables, salads, fresh herbs, spices, sea vegetables, and small amounts of whole grains and fruits. The health of the gut microbiota cannot be underestimated as we age. Every year there is more and more research published demonstrating links between healthy microflora and a healthy weight, immune system, brain, lungs, bones and cardiovascular system.

Data gathered by The British Gut Project indicates that good health throughout life is linked to a greater diversity of microbes in the gastrointestinal tract, and that this is strongly linked to the number of different plant foods that is eaten every week. So aim for at least thirty different **types** of plant foods every week. Once you've built all of this into your diet it will be easier to eat less of the sugars and processed foods that cause havoc in the body and drive inflammaging.

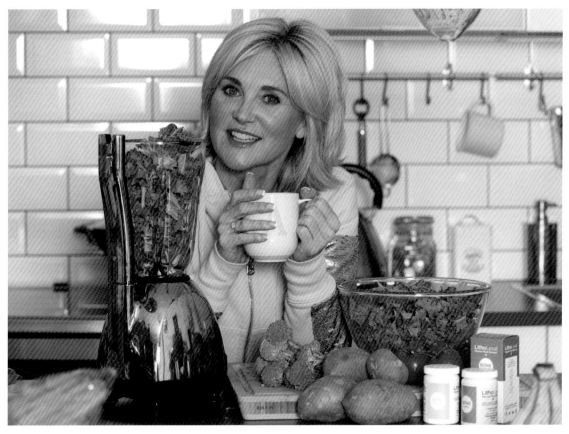

I AIM TO EAT WHOLEFOODS AS MUCH AS POSSIBLE

WHAT ARE THE MOST COMMON PROBLEMS WE EXPERIENCE AS WE AGE?

- Unwanted weight gain, especially around the midriff

- Loss of muscle mass and loss of bone density

- Problems with memory, cognition and a typical symptom is 'brain fog'

- Mood swings, apathy and general low mood, with a feeling of being unable to deal with stress

- Fatigue and in particular mid-afternoon slumps

- Poor sleep: sometimes it may be hard to get to sleep but the more common problem seems to be waking up in the early hours and not being able to get back to sleep

- Lack of temperature control: many women experience feeling too cold all the time; but the very same women can also suffer from hot flashes and night sweats

- Dry skin, dry hair, dry eyes and feeling dry and sore in the urinary-genital area. This can lead to discomfort during sexual intimacy or in some cases even feeling uncomfortable sitting down for too long

- Stiff and sore joints, making it increasingly difficult to maintain motivation for regular exercise

- Gastrointestinal problems such as alternating constipation and diarrhoea, abdominal discomfort, bloating, gas and/or reflux

Many of these symptoms (but not all) are caused or exacerbated by the tendency to increased inflammation as we age, and by hormonal fluctuations (oestrogen and progesterone) typically from the early to mid-forties, and then a sharp decline in these hormones from the late forties or early fifties. And then a deficiency of these hormones for the rest of life. This tends to cause different issues at different ages depending on the stage of the hormonal transition. Thyroid function can also become compromised during mid-life and sometimes it can be hard to differentiate between symptoms that are to do with sex hormone decline and those that are originating from problems with thyroid hormones.

CAN YOU RECOMMEND ANY SUPPLEMENTS FOR MENOPAUSAL WOMEN?

As a baseline, I would say that it is crucial that every woman in mid-life should ensure that she is getting the optimal level of all vitamins and minerals, plant chemicals, amino acids and essential fatty acids that are required for her individual phenotype. (And the phenotype depends on the combination of her genetic inheritance is and the sum total of her life events that will have affected the way her genes work.) So most women in mid-life benefit from a good **multivitamin** and **mineral** supplement, as well as supplemental **omega 3 EPA** and **DHA** (extracted from fish oil, krill or algae), and some extra **magnesium**. Magnesium is hard to get at sufficient levels in the diet and it is needed for more than three hundred different enzymes in the body, so for pretty much every biological process that we need to keep us healthy.

While there are all sorts of other supplements that may be helpful, choosing the right ones can be a bit of a lottery. It might be worth engaging some expert help to analyse your state of health, possibly with the use of laboratory testing, in order to devise a programme of nutritional supplements that is personalised to your individual needs.

WHAT ARE THE MOST COMMON MISCONCEPTIONS WOMEN HAVE ON NUTRITION AND DIETARY NEEDS?

I would say that most people who come to see me for help have already tried to work out how to eat well and have done a lot of their own research. They have often trialled various different ways of eating. So it's not through lack of effort that people may be eating in an unhelpful way for their health. It's really because there is such a lot of confusing information out there and also because eating 'food-like substances' (as opposed to whole, natural foods) has become the norm in society, mainly pushed by manufacturers of processed foods. Hence consumables like white pasta, crusty French bread, processed meats like ham and sausages, fruit juices, breakfast cereals, even salad dressings made with oxidised oils, artificial flavours and added sugars, have all become staples. But if you think about it, they're not real food - they simply have their origin in real food.

Here are some key misconceptions:

- I have to eat every three hours to support my blood sugar levels

- There are a lot of things I can't eat because I am allergic or intolerant to them

- Meat, eggs and dairy are bad for health

- Fruit is healthy and so I eat six or seven pieces a day instead of more 'fattening' foods

- I take a probiotic (live bacteria) every day because that is necessary for good gut health

- Fatty foods are unhealthy and so I cut down on fat as much as possible

- Raw fruits and vegetables are always much healthier than cooked

- It is possible to get all the protein I need from eating vegetables and quinoa

- Nobody should need to take supplements unless they are very ill because everyone can get everything they need from their diet

- I can't eat a lot of vegetables because they make me feel bloated

- I have to be on a low calorie diet and keep track of my calories every day in order to maintain a healthy weight

IS THERE SUCH A THING AS A BAD DIET?

Absolutely! Although there is no such thing as one healthy diet for all, there is plenty of research to show that if we rely too heavily on processed foods rather than food naturally found in nature, we become deficient in the vital life nutrients like vitamins, minerals, phytochemicals, fibre and essential fatty acids. The human body just cannot work well without optimal levels of these. A diet of processed foods also tends to be excessively high in sugars, refined starch and factory made fats, all of which disrupt cellular function and cause disease. What I would say to anyone who doesn't believe me is this: write down how you're feeling right now, including all the niggling symptoms and aches and pains you've been carrying, and how your mood, sleep and energy levels feel to you. Then switch to a healthy diet; in a month's time repeat the diary exercise. How do you feel?

By the way, one way to help with sticking with real foods, is to limit your supermarket shop to certain sections of the store. If you shop only from the inside of the perimeter wall (perhaps the aisle facing that as well) and don't venture into the centre aisles of the supermarket, you will find that your trolley is far fuller of real foods rather than processed food-like substances.

LORRAINE'S TOP NUTRITION TIPS FOR AGEING WELL

- Keep insulin in check: insulin spiking drives inflammation and causes our cells to start rejecting it ('insulin resistance'). Insulin resistance massively increases the risk of almost all age-related diseases.

- Eat food that is real. Ditch anything made in a factory.

- Get loads of plant foods: ten portions of vegetables a day, in as many bright colours as possible, and at least thirty different types of plant foods in the course of one week.

- Don't stint on protein as this becomes even more important for keeping us healthy as we age - without it, our skin, muscles and bones would atrophy, and our brain chemistry, hormones and immune system would struggle to function.

- Human physiology works on a twenty-four-hour clock, which means that our bodies and minds are healthier and happier with regular routines. So eat only during daylight hours, and eat at around the same times every day if you can. No midnight snacking!

- Enjoy your healthy food and make it a shared experience wherever possible.

CAN WE MAINTAIN A HEALTHY WEIGHT AS WE AGE?

Yes we absolutely can. But it's going to be different for everybody because in order to get to an optimal weight you need to identify which body systems are acting as barriers to weight loss, and then work to support these body systems so that they function optimally again and the barriers are removed. For example, once you're eating a healthy diet, you can have a transformational effect on body weight by taking a closer look at the make-up of your gut microbiome, your sex hormone levels, your blood sugar and insulin control mechanisms, your thyroid function, your stress hormone system, your toxic load and detoxification capability, and the functioning of the batteries of your cells (called the mitochondria). Once all of these systems are working well, a good healthy weight is far easier to achieve and maintain.

ARE ALL 'DIETS' FADS OR ARE THERE ANY YOU SUPPORT?

Many 'diets' are fads in that they seem to have no evidence for their benefits and they don't tend to be at all helpful and may even cause harm. For example, it used to be thought that restricting dietary fat as much as possible was the best thing to do for weight loss and overall health. But now we know but that this is a sure-fire way to trigger unwanted weight gain, metabolic imbalances, nutrient deficiencies and loss of control of our appetite!

Nevertheless! there are good reasons why an individual might find it helpful to try certain types of restrictive diets, particularly in the short term. These diets are therapeutic and so by their very nature they are used in order to alter the way body functions work. They are there to make changes within our biochemistry. They are not designed to be followed over the long-term; and generally I would say that most people do well on a more broad-ranging, wholefoods way of eating in the longer-term, as we've already discussed.

Some examples of short-term therapeutic diets that can be powerful, are:

Diets that reduce the level of fermentable carbohydrates where there is an overgrowth of problematic microbes in the gastrointestinal tract, causing gas, bloating and other symptoms.

Diets that restrict carbohydrates generally, and in particular, sugars and concentrated starches like potatoes, sweet potatoes and grains, even whole grains, in order to support individuals who are having trouble with managing their blood glucose levels, especially if they are diabetic or pre-diabetic.

Diets that remove foods that an individual feels worse on when eating. Common such foods are wheat, dairy, beans and pulses. Although most people can tolerate these foods, avoiding them for a while can be hugely helpful for many people who are struggling with their health. The reasons are many and varied but there is no getting away from the fact that those of us who practice nutrition clinically see this time and time again with our clients.

Diets that remove lectins, which are found in many grains, beans and pulses, dairy, nightshade fruits and vegetables, and nuts and seeds. This is a particularly restrictive way of eating but certain individuals, particularly those with autoimmune conditions, can find it beneficial.

Even a truly ketogenic diet can have its place. This is hard to do because to get into ketogenesis you need to be eating mainly fat and not a lot else. But, for example, in certain types of cancers, ketogenic diets can support the efficacy of chemotherapy and may even reduce the side effects of the medical treatment.

Importantly, all these types of diets are designed for short-term use only. They are designed to push pathways in the body and are not supposed to be used as long-term healthy eating programmes. Used appropriately, they can be phenomenally powerful. And while evidence from human trials is lacking, logical mechanisms for their efficacy have been identified in laboratory and animal studies and there is a great deal of unpublished, informal evidence from the clinical practice of nutrition practitioners working in a personalised way."

—— **Lorraine Nicolle** ——

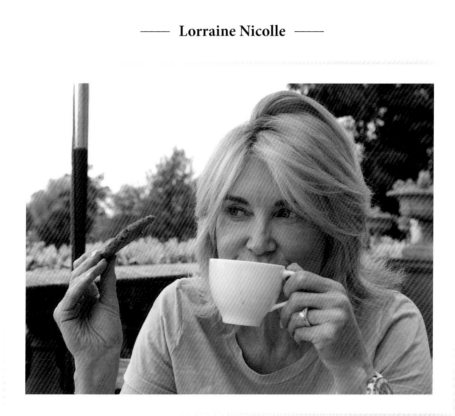

LIKE EVERYONE I ENJOY THE OCCASIONAL TREAT!

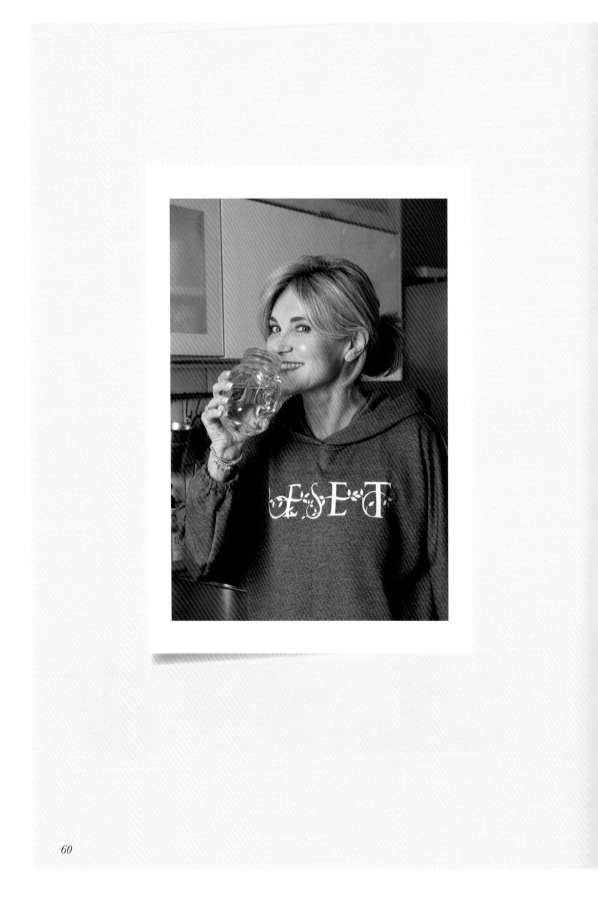

CHAPTER IV

— Gut Health —

I HAD to really start thinking about my diet seriously when I joined *GMTV*. Because first thing in the morning, you haven't got time to sort yourself out. You've got to hit that sofa sparkling, feeling great, and be able to project that down the camera lens to everyone watching from home. I became more aware that the quality of sleep and the quality of food I had, definitely had a direct impact on the way I felt waking up in the morning and doing a job at an ungodly hour. You are paid to look awake, have a sharp mind, lots of energy and glowing skin.

I started in a very rudimentary way, to cut down on meat and eventually I cut it out altogether for about seven years, although I still ate fish. I felt better without so much meat in my diet. (Now I have a balance but at the time I noticed it helped me not to eat it.) So it was really by accident that I started to assess what I was eating because I had a reason to do so. It soon became apparent that eating a banana was going to leave me feeling better than eating a Mars bar!

In those days, no one was talking about gut health but that link with what I ate and how I felt afterwards is exactly that: it's gut health. I've noticed more and more awareness around the issue in the last five years or so, although my friend Liz Earle has been banging on about it for twenty years! She introduced me to **Shann Nix Jones** who talks about looking after the gut, feeding the gut, this amazing mechanism that digests food, that sends it off to the right places in your body…I am certainly not monastic about this, I like a few naughties but I have seen what eating too much of the wrong foods can do to you. I have felt it and I don't want to feel like that again if I can help it.

I am a huge fan of Shann and what she has achieved. She and her husband Rich set up the massively successful business Chuckling Goat which makes the probiotic kefir and other products using goats milk from their farm in Wales after realising how beneficial it was, first when their son was ill and then Rich. This tiny business they developed at their farmhouse table has grown from strength to strength and now they've got more than seventy goats and thousands of customers in nearly thirty countries!

I have a 70ml shot of Chuckling Goat kefir every morning without fail. I prefer it to other kefirs because it's made from goats' milk. I'm not lactose intolerant but I like it. I also have their prebiotic each morning which enhances the effect of the kefir. It comes in powder form which I add to the kefir for speed.

Every time I eat something or drink something, I think: is my gut going to like this? I've made myself like certain things I didn't really used to and I've made some food swaps. For instance, I used to love all chocolate but now I will eat only dark chocolate. I'll have just two squares each night and I don't even like milk chocolate now, it tastes too sweet - yipee! I find that's enough to satisfy my taste buds. I have oat milk rather than dairy and organic wine if possible, instead of non-organic. It's about making better choices a part of my lifestyle. I've found it works for me - for my gut - so I don't feel bloated and tired which I do if I've eaten badly.

— *A* —

"I FIRST learned about gut health to try to help my family, when the doctors couldn't help us. I then fell in love with the fascinating science that demonstrates all the ways that our gut health controls our daily well-being. If you're looking to improve your energy, mood, cognition, sleep, skin or allergies - you can start by improving your gut health. Issues like eczema, IBS, IBD, anxiety, rheumatoid arthritis, fatigue, depression, a weakened immune system - these are all symptomatic leaves of a single tree - and the trunk of that tree sits in your gut.

Imagine your gut like a tiny, exquisite farm, full of living creatures who need to be carefully tended. Your gut bugs are critical for your health - but they also depend on you to maintain them. It's a connected, interdependent relationship. These fragile creatures can easily be damaged by what I call the 'Four Horsemen of the Gut Apocalypse' - sugar, stress, antibiotics and chemicals found in our everyday household cleaners and personal care products.

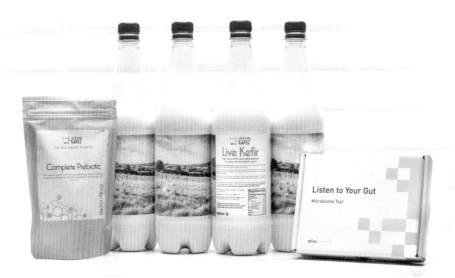

MY CHUCKLING GOAT STAPLES

The simplest way to look after your gut bugs every day is to drink a daily gut health smoothie containing a therapeutic-grade multi-strain probiotic like kefir, which helps boost the strains of healthy bacteria and increase diversity. Then add a scoop of prebiotic fibre, to feed those living bacteria.

Taking a microbiome test is a wonderful way to check the current state of your gut health, and get some evidence-based recommendations on how to improve it. I feel that we're so fortunate to be living in a time when this amazing technology is available on our doorstep, available for our personal use!"

SHANN JONES, FOUNDER AND DIRECTOR CHUCKLING GOAT, GUT HEALTH
EXPERT AND AUTHOR OF THREE BEST SELLING BOOKS ON THE SUBJECT.
www.chucklinggoat.co.uk

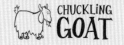

The Gut Health Experts

***

As I've already explained, I started learning about gut health when I had to. What I ate was having an impact on my job because I happened to be working unusual hours and having to look and perform in a certain way and it was imperative I felt as good as I possibly could in order to do a good job.

But many people don't necessarily make the connection because they're too busy getting on with life or it just hasn't popped up on their radar that gut health is vital for our health and general well-being.

Gut health expert, nutritional therapist and health coach **Ailsa Hichens** knows all too well the vital role our digestive system and gut plays in our lives and more so as we age. Here she breaks it down into bitesize pieces…

"IF you don't feel you have anything wrong with your digestion, you might be tempted to skip this section of the book. Don't. Everything about your health depends on your how healthy your gut is. That's not an exaggeration. Your mood, energy, weight, hunger levels, skin, hormonal symptoms like hot flushes, how well you fight illness or disease, and how healthy your heart is. Even your vagina will be more troublesome if the ecology of your digestive system is out of balance. And, of course, if you do struggle with tummy problems, there's that, too.

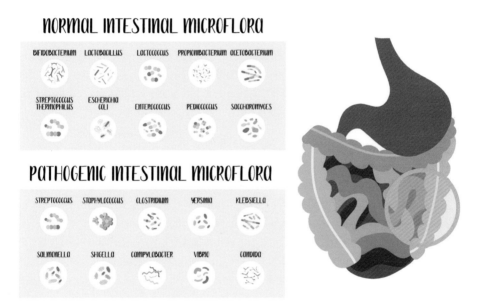

NORMAL INTESTINAL MICROFLORA

BIFIDOBACTERIUM	LACTOBACILLUS	LACTOCOCCUS	PROPIONIBACTERIUM	ACETOBACTERIUM
STREPTOCOCCUS THERMOPHILUS	ESCHERICHIA COLI	ENTEROCOCCUS	PEDIOCOCCUS	SACCHAROMYCES

PATHOGENIC INTESTINAL MICROFLORA

STREPTOCOCCUS	STAPHYLOCOCCUS	CLOSTRIDIUM	YERSINIA	KLEBSIELLA
SALMONELLA	SHIGELLA	CAMPYLOBACTER	VIBRIO	CANDIDA

COURTESY CHUCKLING GOAT

Over the last decade, there has been an explosion of understanding of what we call the 'microbiome' and the impact it has on every aspect of your health. The microbiome is a complex ecosystem made up of a hundred trillion microbes. We call the community of these microbes the 'microbiota', and the community is made up of bacteria, viruses, yeasts, and fungi, most of which live in your gut. Before we talk about this eco system, let's have a think about what your digestive system should be doing. Quick anatomy check-in…

Digestion begins in the brain. I know! When you see, smell or think about food, your appetite is whetted and your saliva flows, which contains digestive enzymes primed and ready to break down the food you're about to eat. It's always a good idea to slow down a bit rather than eating on the go for this very reason.

Your teeth mechanically tear and break down your food. Lots of chewing please so it's a real mush. This creates the greatest surface area so those enzymes and also stomach acid can break the food down further.

That work happens in the stomach after you swallow the food. The stomach acid is also responsible for killing off any bacteria on the food as well as for the absorption of some vitamins.

The resulting slurry then passes to the small intestine, a long, narrow tube that connects the stomach to the large intestine. There's loads of activity going on here – digestive enzymes from the small intestine combine with enzymes from the liver and pancreas to further break apart the nutrients from what you eat and drink so it can be absorbed into your bloodstream.

The large intestine (aka the bowel) is the last part of the digestive system and connects to the anus, where you dump your waste. The large intestine is where water, salts and electrolytes are absorbed from the indigestible food residue.

When we talk about good digestive health, we're talking about this whole process working as it should. When we talk about 'good and bad bacteria' or the microbiome, we mean the bacterial balance in the large intestine – and specifically the part of the large intestine called the cecum.

Now you know all this, you'll have a better understanding of why things can go wrong as you get older.

As you know, all kinds of things work differently (and often not quite as well as they did years ago) as you get older - so why would your digestive system be any different?

Levels of stomach acid start to decline which means your food is not always broken down as well as it might be in the stomach. Since this stomach acid is responsible for breaking down the protein component in your food, where protein is inadequately broken down, it can start to putrefy, causing gas, bloating and inflammation. Ew!

Incidentally, this gas can be the cause of a misdiagnosis of too much stomach acid. Really. What happens is that the pressure caused by putrefaction gasses pushes up the oesophageal flap that keeps the stomach contents in the stomach, and a little stomach acid can pop up, causing the feeling of heartburn. Your natural instinct might then be to pop heartburn remedies or antacids, which just exacerbate the problem, where taking a little tot of apple cider vinegar (choose the one described as 'with mother' not the regular vinegar, which is for your salad dressings) before a meal might be much more beneficial.

At the same time, digestive enzyme production slows, further compromising digestion.

Since food is not being broken down as well, it typically takes longer for it to move through your system, increasing the chance of constipation and irritable bowel syndrome (IBS), along with a host of other unfortunate digestive conditions. And, since the relative lack of stomach acid means less 'bad bacteria' is likely to be killed off, your immune system is also under threat.

MICROBIOME

Let's look again at the microbiome because that changes, too, as we get older. You'll want to listen up because this is what scientists think might hold the key to a longer, healthier and happier life.

This microbiome serves many functions, from breaking down carbohydrates, supporting immunity and detoxification, to producing vitamins, minerals and short-chain fatty acids. Take care of it, and it will take good care of you.

This bacterial environment is never static, and it's been changing unnoticed since the day you were born. Its composition alters both positively and negatively in response to what you put in your body (food, drink, medications or drugs) and your lifestyle (stress and exercise, among others).

Typically, as you get older, your microbiome will look very different to that of a younger person. In fact, scientists can now pretty accurately predict your age based on the make-up of your gut alone.

What happens is that the bacteria become less diverse and some of the most important – like lactobacillus and Bifidobacterium – lose ground in favour of more opportunistic bacteria (think, 'bad' bacteria) that are often the cause of poor health.

One of the things many people fear most about advancing age is brain diseases like Alzheimer's where you literally lose the essence of who you are. Although the scientific community has suspected for a while that the microbiome might hold the answer, now they know for sure. It does. There is a definite link between the bacteria in your gut and development of the disease. Since Alzheimer's is the biggest cause of dementia if you want to hold onto your marbles as you get older, you'll want to take care of your microbiome.

DOWN THERE

As women of a 'certain age', you should also know that there is a big link between your lady hormones and the microbiome. In fact, there is something called the estrobolome, and here's why it's important: the estrobolome is the community of bacteria responsible for metabolising and modulating oestrogen levels in your body. That means your gut bacteria affect your oestrogen levels, which has a big impact on your weight, your sex drive and how you feel along with other pesky symptoms like hot flushes and night sweats, memory problems, and problems with your vagina.

It's all to do with an enzyme called beta glucuronidase, which impacts on the level of oestrogen circulating in the body. This can lead to too much or too little circulating oestrogen and changes in the various different forms of oestrogen. We used to think those menopause-related symptoms were just about the ovaries and what was going on over there but now we know the gut plays a key role. Levels of oestrogen and progesterone affect the hormone receptors in your gut, which dictate how well (or otherwise) your gut works. And an unbalanced gut is terrible news for those menopausal symptoms.

What's more, your microbiome really does affect what's going on 'downstairs'. As you age, your vagina is slowly dying. We call that vaginal atrophy and with it come a host of terrible symptoms, from dryness and discomfort, to increased infections like cystitis, bacterial vaginosis and thrush, pain during sex due to the dryness and also vaginal 'shortening' (that's a lie for a start, think 'shrinking' –

your vagina is the Thumbelina of body parts). So, yes, you must eat, drink and live well most of the time to have a healthy vagina, and a happy, healthy mid-life.

HOW TO EAT WELL FOR A GOOD GUT

Fortunately, there is a lot you can do to start to rebalance your gut. The helpful thing about conversations about nutrition is that many of the same rules apply to gut health as they do to other areas of your health.

Number one is that sugar is not your friend. You might have a real taste for it or even be hooked on it since sugar is a hidden ingredient in many foods, but it is disastrous for the gut.

Here's the truth: the effects of a poor diet are mediated by your microbiome. If that is out of whack, there is literally no back-up plan. The science shows us that a high-sugar diet creates an environment where opportunistic (think 'bad') bacteria can run riot, while also decreasing abundance of the 'good' bacteria. This in turn has an impact on inflammation levels and on the integrity of the gut. The latter describes how permeable your gut is. It's supposed to be selectively permeable so that nutrients can get out into the bloodstream but too far in the wrong direction (aka 'leaky gut') and you're at risk of problems like food intolerances and autoimmune conditions.

SUGAR IS THE ENEMY!

Stop the damage now by cutting right back on sugar. There are so many reasons to do this – like energy and hormone balance to name just a couple – but rebalancing your gut is a good enough reason to take action. For similar reasons, steer clear of refined carbohydrates like bread, pastries, cakes and biscuits, and other products made with white flour where the beneficial fibre content has been removed or changed.

Many of these products contain a protein called gluten, which is found in grains like wheat, barley and rye. There's a lot of talk about the effect of gluten on digestive health, with many (including myself) standing by the literature that suggests gluten is bad news since it may lead to leaky gut syndrome, while others (including the NHS) claiming the evidence is not compelling enough.

There are studies that show that gluten activates something called zonulin, which is the regulator of intestinal permeability, causing the normally tight junctions in the gut to slacken such that particles you don't want in your bloodstream escape and wreak havoc.

Personally, I wouldn't chance it. When you follow an unrefined, wholefood diet, you'll be cutting out a lot of gluten anyway and options for going gluten-free if you're out and about are plentiful.

WHOLEFOODS

So then, we're back to eating real food. For digestive health, that means eating a diverse diet to feed your microbes. A healthy gut has a diverse community of microbes and they all like something different for dinner. Although everyone is different, the following is a good general guideline:

Base your meals around the concept of a Mediterranean diet, which does not mean eating the kind of foods you would find in your local Italian restaurant. The typical 'Western diet', featuring a lot of red and processed meat, fried foods, high-fat dairy products, potatoes, and sweetened drink, is not conducive to a healthy gut environment.

Instead, focus on eating more plant-based foods, such as fruit and veggies, pulses like beans, lentils and chickpeas, and wholegrains (think brown rice and wholemeal bread where the whole grain is used).

Aside from any other health benefits (of which there are many), all these foods are rich in fibre, which feed the good bacteria in your gut. These good bacteria then go on to make short-chain fatty acids, which are the main source of energy for the cells lining your colon.

Eating foods containing inulin (garlic, leeks, onions, artichokes, asparagus), fructooligosaccharides aka FOS (onions, garlic, asparagus, bananas), and pectin (apples, carrots, oranges, apricots) are also helpful for encouraging the production of these short-chain fatty acids. When I'm working with my private clients, my advice is to not over-think it.

Focus on trying to get as many fibre-rich foods and different coloured veggies into your diet as you can without feeling you need a checklist.

PROBIOTICS

Eat probiotic foods to help add more 'good' bacteria to the gut. These are foods that contain live bacteria and can improve your microbiome. The one you'll definitely have heard of is 'live' or probiotic yoghurt, which is in every supermarket dairy aisle.

There is a huge variety of probiotic products on offer and, obviously, some are far better than others. As a general rule, steer clear of sweetened yoghurt drinks with added probiotic cultures – some are as sweet as soft drinks to make them palatable. So, with one hand you give but with another, you take away…

The ancient practice of fermenting foods is a winner for digestive health, and there will be some names you may not have heard of. If you're after a tasty probiotic drink, I recommend kefir (a cultured dairy product, although you can also find it made with non-dairy milks) and kombucha (fermented tea). Both are available in the chilled section of many supermarkets, and they taste delicious. Others include sauerkraut and kimchi (fermented cabbage) – both of which are great fun to make at home – and miso, tempeh and natto (made from fermented soy). While once the preserve of health food stores, you'll now find these in the vegan and world food aisles in your local supermarket. I'm not going to lie, they are an acquired taste.

There's even an argument (though not much science behind it), that sourdough bread – fermented slowly using a wide range of bacteria compared to the quickly fermented single strains used in most commercial breads – is easier to digest than regular bread. Logically, it might be that the longer fermentation has begun to break down some of the proteins that might otherwise cause digestive problems. Try it and see if you notice a difference between that and regular bread.

PREBIOTICS

If you've heard of probiotics, you'll likely have also heard of prebiotics. They both relate to bacteria in the gut but do you know the difference? Think of probiotics as adding extra good bacteria. Prebiotics are plant-based foods that make it to the intestines mostly undigested and they feed the bacteria that is there. Imagine the double whammy of combining probiotic with prebiotic foods – that's one of the things that makes overnight oats with natural probiotic yoghurt such a winner.

You might be thinking that prebiotics are always an excellent addition to your diet but hold your horses…

As you get older and that stomach acid I was talking about earlier diminishes and this means that bacteria isn't always killed off and it can end up in places you don't want it. When we talk about 'gut bacteria' we're talking about bacteria in the large intestine. You don't really want any in the small intestine at all and, for various reasons, the daily swoosh of bacteria down to the large intestine (officially called the Migrating Motor Complex) doesn't always work, leaving behind bacteria that feast on the food you're eating. Bacteria here [in the small intestine] can create gasses, and it's these unwanted gasses that lurk behind many cases of IBS and tricky digestive symptoms like gurgling, bloating, belching, diarrhoea and constipation (or alternating bowel movements). Since prebiotics feed bacteria (and you don't get to pick the ones are being fed), prebiotic foods can make uncomfortable digestive symptoms worse.

These are the inulin and FOS foods I mentioned above – and onions and garlic are among the most troublesome - but you can also add to the list the other enemies of the gut: sugar and refined carbs.

Some prebiotic foods seem to be better tolerated by people with digestive issues, including oats (high in beneficial beta glucans) and berries. **You know your body and are the best judge of what agrees with you – or not.**

There are plenty of other prebiotic veggies that have something to bring to the table. I am a fan of smelly vegetables for assorted reasons. Pretty much all veggies that smell contain glucosinolates – the sulphur-containing compounds found in cruciferous veg (this is what gives them the distinctive smell). These glucosinolates are fermented by bacteria and used as fuel. You'll find them in broccoli, brussel sprouts, cauliflower, bok choy, kale, spring greens (aka collard greens in the States), rocket, radishes and cabbage.

If you know your diet is low in fibre generally, now is a great day to start increasing it but know your limits. You will want to increase fibre slowly over a few weeks to allow your body to adjust.

FIVE EASY TIPS THAT ACTUALLY WORK:

There are some even more basic things you can do to enhance digestion and improve your gut. Warning: you will have heard of all of these. Reality check: how often to you actually do them?

1. Take time out for your meals. Appreciate what you are eating, which stimulates saliva in which there are digestive enzymes. This will give you a head start.

2. Eat mindfully. Don't be in a hurry to get the meal done. This works against you in a number of ways - you can't expect good digestion but also eating quicker usually means more mindless eating (and for that, read, potentially, overeating).

3. Chew properly. Your stomach doesn't have teeth. You want to create the biggest surface area for the stomach acid and digestive enzymes to get to work.

4. Struggling with your digestion? Start with food – apple cider vinegar with mother, diluted in a little water, before a meal can help. Then consider supplements.

5. Take a gentle walk after a big meal to help with digestion. Granny was right all along. It really can help.

SUPPLEMENTS FOR GUT HEALTH

Given the extent to which your microbiome – your gut environment – directs and controls your health, you might be wondering whether you can just pop a pill. While eating a diet based on real food is the first strategy you should employ, it can be a good idea to take a supplement for a belt and braces approach.

Start with a probiotic supplement – a capsule rather than one of those sugary drinks. I'd choose one **without any prebiotics if you have any digestive symptoms**. The most common families of bacteria used in probiotics are lactobacillus (as an aside, lactobacillus will be the predominant species in a healthy vagina) and Bifidobacterium.

Each family contains specific strains. Some of the best researched and most beneficial are l. acidophilus, l. rhamnosus, l. reuteri and l.plantarum, and, for the Bifidobacterium, b. animalis, b. infantis, b. lactis, and b. longum. If you struggle with digestive problems, it is best to talk to a qualified professional who can advise as different strains of bacteria can be helpful in supporting different conditions.

However, as a general rule, go for a probiotic that contains a balance of lactobacillus and Bifidobacteria. The amount of bacteria is measured in billions of colony forming units or CFU – essentially the number of viable bacteria. On labels, it might be shown as 1 x 106 or ten billion CFU. The numbers in probiotic supplements usually range from 1 to 50 – or more - billion CFU but there's no hard rule that the more the better. Try to go for a brand that includes a few different strains of the lactobacillus and Bifidobacteria, and steer clear of fillers that might include lactose or corn starch that may cause unpleasant effects, like gas and bloating. If you're looking for one for general digestive health, go for one that will give you at least thirty billion CFU over the day and take on an empty stomach so it has the best chance of arriving where you need it intact without being damaged by your stomach acid. Look for companies to buy from that use very well researched strains and can demonstrate it. This is one area where quality really does matter.

Saccharomyces boulardii, which is actually a beneficial yeast, can also be helpful in redressing balance and improving bowel function, and is helpful to take alongside a daily probiotic to support short-chain fatty acid production and the removal of 'bad' bacteria.

Digestive enzymes are also a great addition, given your body reduces its own natural production with advancing years. They are important because they also help your body absorb the nutrients in your food. Although some folk say, 'you are what you eat' the truth is that you are what you actually absorb.

Some foods contain digestive enzymes naturally – like pineapple, papaya, mango, kiwi, honey, bananas and avocado – a supplement may give you the relief you are looking for if you've already tried the food-first approach.

Digestive enzymes are usually plant-based, and contain the enzymes needed to break down carbs (amylase), fat (lipase), and protein (protease). Most supplements will contain other enzymes, including lactase, which can help you digest dairy products better. As they are designed to mimic your own enzymes, you'll take one just before a main meal. Some are also available with added hydrochloric acid (HCl), which is the same type of acid as your stomach acid. You can buy them wherever you get your supplements.

If you subscribe to the notion that the gut can become inflamed and damage through poor diet, environmental factors, stress and medications and you experience allergies, intolerances, asthma, eczema and other symptoms linked to intestinal permeability (aka gut hyperpermeability - leaky gut) or if you have an autoimmune condition, it may be worth exploring supplements that can be helpful for promoting gut healing, like omega 3 fatty acids, glutamine, collagen, and slippery elm".

—— **Ailsa Hichens** ——

HELPFUL READING

THE CLEVER GUTS DIET: Michael Mosely

THE PIOPPI DIET: Dr Aseem Malhotra & Donal O'Neill

THE HARCOMBE DIET 3-STEP PLAN: Dr Zoe Harcombe

THE KEFIR SOLUTION: Shann Nix Jones

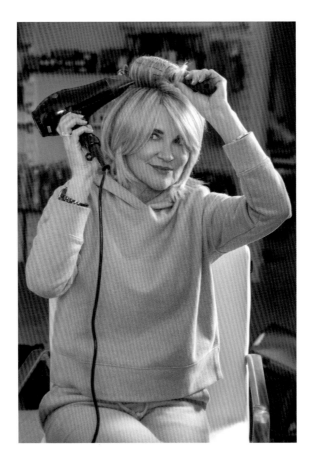

CHAPTER V

— Our Crowning Glory —

AS for every woman, my hair is very important to me. If I'm having a bad hair day, I'm not happy. I'm sure everyone reading this can relate to that. A good haircut and blow-dry can make all the difference to your confidence; it is after all, our crowning glory.

I really believe a good hairstyle can change your life. It makes a huge difference to the way you feel about yourself. The best piece of advice I like to give somebody who asks is stand up straight and smile. But if you don't feel good about yourself, it's very difficult to do.

As I've got older I've learned what suits me and what doesn't. I've also noticed changes in the texture and density of my hair. I know I have a lot of it but I also take care of it in the best way I know how by eating well, taking supplements and not over styling it.

I have naturally curly hair but over the years, with the onset of grey, I'd now refer to it as wavy - remember the seventies' beachcomer look? Well that's me but even that takes a little 'curating'.

If I'm at home and have time, I run a little conditioner through my hair, get on with chores for an hour or so then jump in the shower and wash my hair without reconditioning. Nicky Clarke taught me this trick and it works as conditioner can be counter productive to keeping your bounce. Most people are a little heavy-handed with it; you really need very little.

People don't believe I've ever changed my hairstyle but I actually have! It's just a variation on a layered cut. My hair doesn't suit me all one length, it looks ridiculous. I have no crown so I have a lot of hair on top with lots of layers to give me a shape. It's largely down to my amazing hair dresser **Lino Carbosiero**. I've gone to him for years and I always say I'd never live abroad because I couldn't be without him!

Lino knows my hair as well as I do. He gives me plenty of layers and volume and it enables me to look after my hair myself once I get home. I think that's really important: there's no point in having an elaborate hair style in the salon which you then can't maintain. Lino always says it's vital to get your hair done according to your own personal lifestyle which is so true.

— *A* —

Lino began his career aged just sixteen and has gone on to become one of the UK's most successful celebrity hairdressers counting Kylie Minogue, Jason Donovan, Adel, Jane Horrocks and even Melania Trump among his clientele. And of course yours truly!

After opening his own salon in London in 1985, he joined the exclusive Daniel Galvin salon in 1993 from where he loves nothing better than making his clients feel incredibly special. I've personally been a client – and now a friend – of Lino's for nearly twenty-five years and there's no one I trust more to take care of my hair.

Here are some of his pearls of wisdom when it comes to our hair as we age:

"THE first thing that you notice as we get older is a change of texture in the hair. It can get coarse and quite dry, especially if it's very grey. Hair colour changes also as we age and the amount of hair you have decreases, especially around the front where it's first noticeable.

This can be depressing but it doesn't need to be. The first thing I do with my clients is to deflect from any hair loss. I've got so many clients who have one form of alopecia or another but not necessarily in places they can see. I make sure I cut and style it to cover thin patches. I also offer them advice on the best way of looking after their hair.

I know Anthea worried about her hair at one time and she did something about it. She moisturised it better and ate better and now it's pretty much back to what it was. She does have amazing hair but she also works hard to keep it looking good. She knows how to look after it properly.

It's essential to look after your hair and look after yourself. I always say to my clients, if you have dry skin, what would you do? And they all without exception say they would moisturise it. But I wouldn't say that ten out of ten women would take the same care with their hair. It's vital to look after your hair inside and out. If you eat well and use good products, you will have healthy hair. If you eat fast food every day it's going to catch up with you.

When I say good products, I don't necessarily mean expensive products. If you don't have a good hairdresser to advise you, there are so many products on the market to choose from which don't cost a fortune. It's a case of trial and error to find what works best for you.

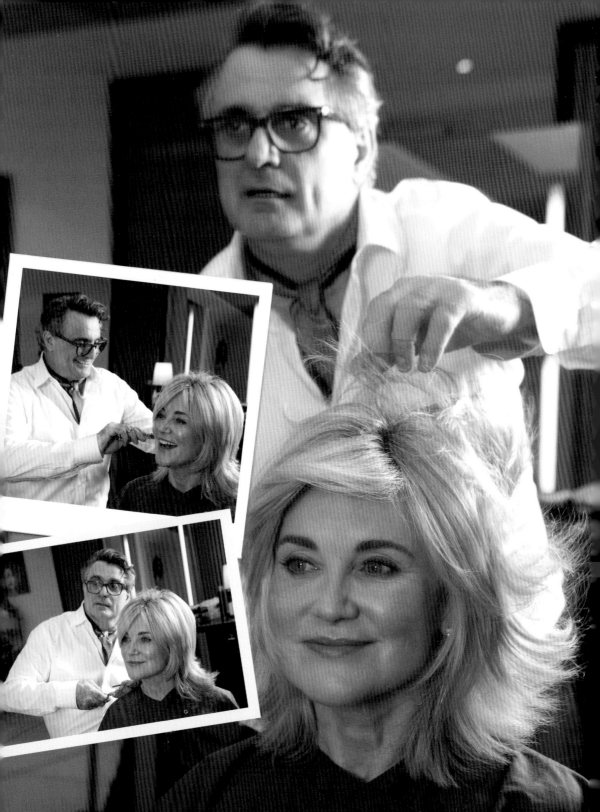

LINO WORKS HIS MAGIC ON MY LOCKS AT DANIEL GALVIN, LONDON

HAIRDRESSER

I would encourage every woman to take advice from her hairdresser. An experienced hairdresser, especially one who has a good relationship with their client, won't be doing the job just for the money. You get to a certain level in this industry where it's literally all about looking after your clients. I must see around eighty different people a week, both men and women. Many are now in their seventies and eighties and have been coming to me for decades. We've learned to trust each other and they know I will always look after them. After lockdown, these were the first people to walk through the door when the salon reopened.

Can I just say, your hairdresser needs help in helping you to achieve the look you want; we can't read minds. In the old days, women would bring in a video for me to watch at home saying, 'This is how I want my hair!' Now you can just bring in a photograph, even if it's the back of someone's head and we can use that to help you. From there we can advise you on what will look best. Sometimes I have to tell my clients this style won't work on you but we could do this, this and this and compromise so you have the style that works best for you. A woman's style has to reflect her lifestyle and the image she wants to portray. A good stylist will listen and help you achieve that.

LONG HAIR?

There's no reason why a woman in her later years has to have short hair. Those days have gone. What really works for me as long as hair has shape and a softness, you can definitely go longer. But if your hair is dragging down and just hanging, it can be very ageing. You can make longer hair look great with fringes or layering. We have to take everything into consideration as women age. Their hairline may recede and will need to be disguised or they may lose volume and texture. That's why a good hairdresser is so important.

GOING GREY?

As you go grey, your hair won't take colour the same way it did when you were younger. You're not going to get the same tones as you did when you first started colouring your hair. You can end up going so dark it can really make you look older than you want to. Skin tones change as we age and having hair too dark can make you look like a ghost.

Covid changed a lot of people's mind-set on this issue. They didn't get their hair coloured during lockdown because they couldn't and they realised it actually didn't matter; they embraced the grey. They weren't going anywhere and they discovered it wasn't so bad. Maybe this will change in future; it will be interesting to see. Personally I love grey hair. There are certain ladies on whom grey hair looks amazing. And it's less hassle.

> Your hair frames your face and should be treated well.
> Would you buy a beautiful painting and stick it in a rubbish frame?

Lino Carbosiero

IT'S GOOD TO LOOK GOOD

There are women who I see who are embarrassed about taking time and trouble over their hair. They think they appear vain. Why? It's like anything else, you have to look after yourself to feel your best. If you look after yourself, you can look after others. You are worth the investment."

***

LINO'S HAIR HACKS:

Make sure you know what's been put in your hair. For example, if you've had it chemically straightened or coloured, the chemicals will be there years later and can affect ongoing treatments. Be hair aware.

As you get older, soften your hair colour and soften the cut. Layers are the way to go. Lots of layers. A good haircut and colour can give you a twinkle in the eye. I tend to advise highlights. Once you commit to having an all-over colour it's an upkeep, it's expensive.

Steer clear of hair extensions. Hair extensions break hair, especially as it ages. If you've got an event and want a dramatic one-off change, I'd recommend clip-in extensions or a hairpiece but never, ever long-term.

Don't over blow-dry your hair. It's really important. If you have to use heated appliances like irons or rollers you must nourish your hair afterwards.

Look after your scalp as well as your hair. There are plenty of scalp treatments on the market but beware of products with silicone in. They will build up and clog up the pores.

On holiday, if you have naturally curly hair, don't wash it every day. Rinse it with water and condition. And if you're at the beach, take a bottle of conditioner with you. Go into the sea, come out and rub a bit of conditioner through your hair and sunbathe that way.

Everyone should wear a hat to protect the hair. After swimming, by the pool or on the beach, if you're not vain then cover up with a plastic cap or even cling film. It's a great treatment.

Don't overuse hair spray. It's difficult to wash out and will form a film, which look like little white specs on the hair when it is next blow dried.

—— **Lino Carbosiero MBE** ——

While Lino does a great job cutting my hair, the wonderful **Wendy Nixon** who owns Armstrong Cuthbert salon in West London, has been colouring my hair for years. She's got decades of experience and knows exactly what works for all her clients, including me.

Here are some of Wendy's thoughts when it comes to colouring our hair as we get older…

"LET'S start with a few home truths. Hair ages just like skin, and as this happens you need to change your hair care products, just as you would your moisturiser or skin cream. As this process happens, thinning, frailty and dullness are common problems we experience, as well as those dreaded greys! The good news is that there are a host of products and routines you can use to counteract these changes. Aveda for example, which we use at Armstrong Cuthbert, have a specific range of products for thinning hair called Invati, a botanical repair range for brittleness and also a colour conserve range. In-salon treatments are also strongly recommended when undergoing a colour treatment, as these can nourish and condition previously lifeless hair. The reason I partnered with Aveda some years ago, is that all their hair products are created from natural ingredients and sustainably sourced. Using the right shampoos/conditioners and visiting your salon a little more often will reap benefits for years to come.

THE DREADED GREYS!

As grey hair sets in (as it does for most), many of us can panic about whether to hide it or manage the situation. Do not be afraid – allowing yourself to go grey naturally is possible with good colour and conditioning treatments that will give your hair lustre. Likewise, if you choose to hide the greys, getting the right shade is key to a natural look that can be finessed over time.

Whichever product range your salon uses, a thorough consultation is a must, so you can agree a detailed plan of how you want to manage your hair moving forwards and which shampoos, conditioners and treatments will best facilitate this.

ANTHEA'S HAIR

When Anthea first came into the salon around five years ago, her hair had bleached highlights and was not in the best condition – I'm sure she won't mind me saying! With her agreement, I added a more natural base colour to add warmth to her skin tone and frame her face more vibrantly. I have also added tint and enlightener to produce creamy blonde highlights and a botanical repair treatment that protects and rebuilds the bonds that can break during the colour process. The result is natural, warm and younger looking, healthy hair.

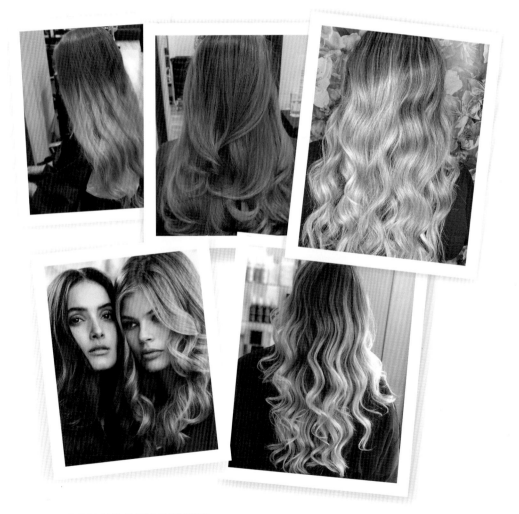

A GOOD HAIR COLOUR SHOULD BE FUN!

DO

- Make sure you have a full consultation with your stylist to agree your hair care plan

- Use regular treatments on your hair, either in-salon or treat yourself at home

- Ensure you undergo an allergy test every six months – your sensitivity can change over time

- Use special sun protection shampoos and conditioners if going on holiday

- Have a clear gloss treatment to add lustre and shine to your hair

- Make regular, small colour changes to keep your look updated as the grey increases

DON'T

- Keep using the same colour you always have! Generally speaking, you need to go lighter in shade as you get older

- Try and do the colour yourself – this rarely ends well and overlapping can result in the hair appearing too dark. It can also be expensive and time consuming to sort out!

- Use overheated styling tools and straighteners, as your hair will get damaged and break

- Have your roots redone and have the colour taken through to the ends every time, as this will make it more brittle and will layer the colour, creating bands; have a colour gloss instead to refresh the ends

TO SUM UP

I have been helping women to stay looking young for many years and there really is no magic formula, just some simple rules to follow. Use good quality aftercare products (shampoos and conditioners) between appointments, have regular haircuts to keep your style strong and make regular small changes to keep your look up to date. As I alluded to earlier, look after your hair as much as you would your skin and take advice from your trusted haircare professional.

Finally, I encourage my clients to take a wider, holistic approach. Diet, smoking and hormone changes can all significantly affect hair quality, so addressing each of these in a positive way will dramatically help you on your haircare journey moving forward".

—— **Wendy Nixon** ——

Brand President and Consultant Trichologist **Anabel Kingsley** at Philip Kingsley explains the science behind our hair as we age. She and her team at the renowned Philip Kingsley clinics, treat hundreds of women - and men - each week, struggling with a number of hair problems, from hair loss to scalp infections:

"EVERYONE'S hair changes as they get older, just as everyone's skin changes as they age. All women can therefore expect a certain amount of density changes because hair follicles start to produce hairs that are not as good quality as they used to be. For some women this is really minimal, but for others density changes can be very noticeable. The degree to which your hair changes is due in large part to genetics.

Density changes leading up to, during and after menopause are largely dependent on whether hair follicles on your scalp have a genetic sensitivity to normal levels of circulating androgens (male hormones). Leading up to the menopause, oestrogen levels start to decline. Oestrogen helps to prolong the growth (anagen) phase of the hair growth cycle. It also acts as a buffer against the effects of testosterone – which can shorten the anagen phase and cause hair follicles to gradually miniaturize and produce finer, shorter strands. Even though testosterone levels don't rise as you get older, the protection that your hair follicles have against testosterone decreases. So if you have this genetic sensitivity where hair follicles on your scalp are sensitive to testosterone, that drop in oestrogen can trigger some quite noticeable density changes. It's called **androgenic alopecia** and it can happen at any age after puberty.

HAIR LOSS

There are many types of hair loss. As I've already mentioned, there's **androgenic alopecia** which is more commonly known as female pattern hair loss or thinning. Contrary to popular belief, this is really common in women. Then you have excessive hair shedding, called telogen effluvium. This is completely different and is not due to genes. Telogen effluvium can happen at any age and is often due to diet, lifestyle, nutritional deficiencies, thyroid imbalances, stress and certain medications. It can also be brought on by hormonal shift so women may initially experience heavy hair shedding when they enter menopause, and also intermittently as their hormone levels continue to change. When hormone levels even out, hair shedding almost always slows down. There are lots of types of hair loss but these two are the main ones that affect women.

DEALING WITH HAIR LOSS

There's no such thing as a hair loss shampoo and I get really upset when I see brands promoting a shampoo promising that it's going to stop your hair falling out. Even if a shampoo contains all the right ingredients, it isn't left on your scalp long enough for those actives to have an impact on your hair growth cycle in the way they need to. This is why things like prescribed scalp drops containing actives such as Minoxidil or another stimulant mixed with an anti-androgen are good because they stay on for an extended period of time. What does help is regular shampooing because it keeps your scalp healthy. Your scalp is your hair support system. Your scalp is also skin and should be cleansed regularly, just as you cleanse the skin on your face regularly. If you have dandruff, clearing that up with anti-dandruff shampoo can help. Research has proven a flaky scalp can contribute to hair shedding.

CARING FOR OUR HAIR AS WE AGE

In terms of growing your healthiest head of hair as you grow older, diet and lifestyle are so important. So if you are not eating a well-balanced varied diet, getting all the vitamins and minerals and trace nutrients you need, your hair is going to suffer basically because it's not an essential tissue. This means that whenever you're not eating well, your hair cell production is the first place your body diverts its attention away from. Your hair cells are the second fastest growing cells your body produces so they're really needy. Complex carbohydrates provide slow, accessible release of energy to your body. Proteins are needed because your hair is made of protein; they are used to build tissue like your hair.

You should also take care of the condition of your hair externally. If your hair has become finer, it will be more fragile and will break under less force. As well as this, you may be colouring your hair more, which can also weaken and dry it out. This means it's important to use intensive products that both strengthen and moisturise. I love our Elasticizer pre-shampoo conditioner, which my father formulated for Audrey Hepburn, and our Bond Builder Re-Structuring Treatment. Also, treat your hair with care; be gentle when you style and brush and use a low to medium heat setting on your dryer. Daily wear and tear can really take its toll on your strands.

SUPPLEMENTS

Supplements are meant to supplement a healthy diet. They will only help if your hair is coming out because you're not getting the nutrients you need which I must say is quite common because your hair's nutritional requirements are very high. If you know which areas you're deficient in, you can choose the exact supplement/s you need. If you want to be specific, get a blood test to see if and where there are any deficiencies. For instance, iron and ferritin (stored iron) deficiency are very common, especially if you're still losing blood each month or have heavy periods. Don't be tempted to analyse your results yourself – numbers cannot be viewed in isolation and, as hair is non-essential tissue, the blood reference range for optimal hair growth is different than for optimal general health.

We do a really good supplement at Philip Kingsley which we've based on the tens of thousands of blood tests that we've analysed over the years. From these, we know what the most common nutritional deficiencies are, and the amount of each nutrient needed by most women. We have something called **Tricho Complex Hair Nutrition Supplement** which has iron, vitamin C which is needed for iron absorption, l-lysine which is needed for iron storage, vitamin D, Biotin and vitamin B12. Then we have a separate protein supplement which helps give your hair the protein it needs. Those are retail, you don't need a prescription.

WELL-BEING

I lost my hair when my father passed away and again post-partum. I also have a chronic health condition which when it flares up, causes my hair to fall out. So I know from personal experience it can be absolutely debilitating even if you know why it's happening and what you have to do to fix it. I've had women who are very tearful, some who are actually suicidal. Hair is not just hair. It's part of our identity as women. A lot of my clients say 'My hair is my thing.' Hair is everyone's thing, whether it's the colour or the cut. It's linked to who we are so when we lose it, it's like losing a part of ourselves.

GET HELP SOONER RATHER THAN LATER

It's really difficult for women to look for solutions as female hair loss is still such a taboo subject and I feel like women often suffer in silence and leave it far too long to seek help. They believe they're the only ones going through it or they're embarrassed or there's too much information and there are too many brands and companies promising x, y and z. I'm not saying this to get people into our Clinic. We are not an inexpensive service but I think a lot of women will try several less costly options first, going for a product they saw online or Instagram or that their hairdresser suggested. So a year passes by with them using all these solutions that are promising amazing results which never materialise. Female pattern hair loss is particularly progressive so then you've wasted a year. I'd say do your research and go to the experts from the beginning. It's not too late but it is slightly more difficult the longer you leave it to seek help. You've also suffered unnecessarily and wasted a lot of money.

DYE

Permanent hair dyes are always going to be more damaging than semi-permanent or temporary dyes but you're never going to have the same aesthetic result as a permanent colour. I'd say simply go to a hairdresser you trust and who knows what your hair can take. Hair is here for us to have fun with it so if you want to be blonde, redhead or brunette and it makes you feel better, go ahead and do it but just make sure it's something your hair can withstand. Hair extensions are different as they can cause hair loss or **traction alopecia**. I say to people it's fine if you're going to a special event: buy some really good clip in extensions but don't get permanent ones put in. It's just disguising any hair loss and it's also causing hair loss. I don't recommend permanent extensions. Ever. "

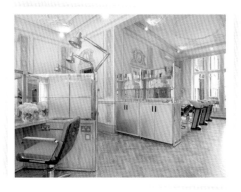

©PHILIP KINGSLEY

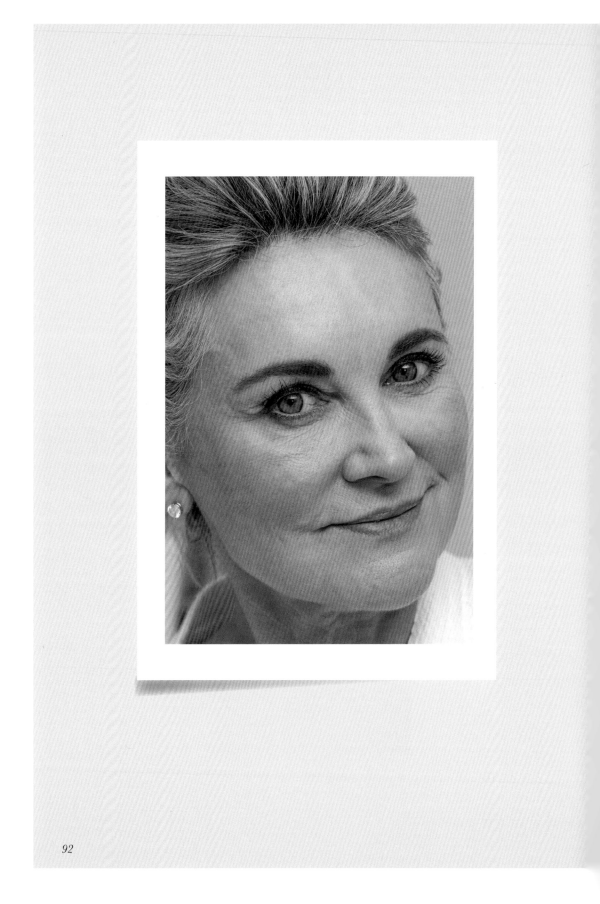

CHAPTER VI

— *Skin* —

I WAS very unlucky – and lucky – that in 1988 I had an accident while presenting Saturday morning telly with a pyrotechnic that went off in my face. It was bad enough to take me off television for a couple of weeks but not bad enough to scar my skin.

During the escapade, I went off to see – on the insistence of Gloria Hunniford – a plastic surgeon by the name of Dev Basra who gave me the best advice anyone could have given me. I remember saying to him, 'I'll just sit outside and let the sun mend my skin.' He replied, 'You do that, you will have pigmentation problems for the rest of your life. I'd tell you this even if you hadn't burnt your face; for the rest of your life, keep out of the sun as much as possible and use a high SPF on your skin every single day.'

From then on I think I've had a reasonably good relationship with the sun and while I love a sunny holiday as much as the next person, I always make sure I don't overdo it. I wear lots of skin protection and don't sunbathe for long. I'm more worried about sun damage now than I've ever been yet last year, I had the best tan I've ever had. I used factor 50 on my face and factor 30 everywhere else and still managed to achieve a lovely, healthy glow which lasted a long time. However, I could have done better. I do have sunspots which annoy me but I have to remember each one represents an imense amount of travelling which included, sailing, horse riding and a damn good time!

Apart from sun damage, a poor diet and lack of exercise can adversely impact the skin which I'm very aware of. We're all born with a lovely, healthy skin and then slowly through bad habits like smoking, drinking too much alcohol, too much sun exposure, a bad diet and so on, it is destroyed. Then somewhere in our forties, we wake up to this destruction and notice the pigmentation spots, the lines which have arrived too early and the wrinkles which have appeared from seemingly nowhere.

You can't really reverse the damage but it's never too late to tweak and make certain changes. You can improve and help your skin from the inside out. I watch my diet, I don't drink a lot and I exercise. I also take a collagen supplement every single day and swear by it. There are lots of brands that make it but the one I use is by Rejuvenated which was founded by the wonderful **Kathryn Danzy** who strongly believes beauty and well-being starts from within. My friend **Grace Foder** (see also Chapter IX Style) introduced us about six years ago because she knew I'd love what she had to say.

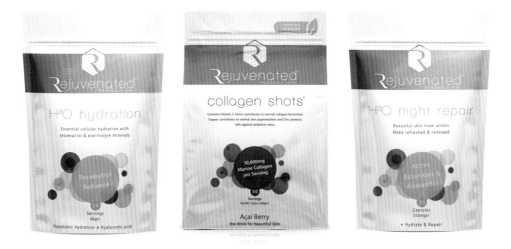

REJUVENATED PRODUCTS I TAKE REGULARLY FOR MY SKIN

Kathryn, with her family, has developed a whole range of supplements, some of which I now won't be without as they're amazing for my skin. I am particularly hooked on Rejuvenated's Collagen Shots which has won several awards so I'm not the only one who agrees it's fabulous! It's jam-packed with marine extract collagen, antioxidant-rich acai berry, hyaluronic acid plus Vitamins B and C. Collagen supports your extracellular tissue throughout the body. As Kathryn herself points out, 'The really surprising thing is that collagen is in so much more than the skin; you can find it in your joints, muscles, bones, digestive system, hair, nails, heart and brain.'

I also use Rejuvenated's H30 Hydration and H30 Night Repair supplements. www.rejuvenated.com

My skincare routine is pretty simple. I'm religious about cleansing at night, I exfoliate properly about once a week and am obsessed by a vitamin C serum I get from **Dr Andrew Weber** (who you can read more about in Chapter VIII Nip and Tuck).

I've discovered as you get older you need products containing the big guns and they do make a difference. So when shopping around I look for products which include retinol, vitamins A, C,and E as well as hyaluronic acid and tretinoin.

But whatever the weather I use a sunscreen on my face neck and back of hands.

I'm a great believer in trying out different products and treatments which I can do because I'm not on anyone's payroll. Everyone has to find out what works best for them but when I find something I'm genuinely pleased with, I am happy to share it with others. I also tend to stick with things that work for me.

— *A* —

Like all women of my age, I've noticed changes in my skin, especially in the last ten years. As I've already explained, I keep out of the sun as much as I can, use the best products I can afford and stick to a healthy diet.

I don't have many break-outs (although with the menopause and fluctuating hormones, I have had my share of problems in the past) but many women do experience various skin issues at different stages of their lives and need specialist help.

Of course your own GP can refer you to a dermatologist if you need one but if you're looking for a recommendation, the excellent **Dr Emma Wedgeworth** at Dr Sam Bunting's Clinic in London is your woman. She specialises in all skin problems including sun damage and acne and believes in a holistic lifestyle approach to achieving gorgeous skin.

Here she explains how our skin changes as we age and how we can achieve something every woman wants – great looking skin!

"OVER the years, profound changes happen to our skin at all levels. The outer layer of our skin – known as our skin barrier - becomes weaker and our skin becomes more sensitive. Pigmentation becomes more uneven with the appearance of sun spots. Deeper down, collagen (one of the main structural proteins in our skin) reduces in quantity and in quality, which leads to the appearance of lines and wrinkles. The elasticity of our skin also reduces and we lose fat in our face, both of which contribute to sagging and volume loss.

The eye area is one of the first to show signs of ageing, because the skin here is so thin. Fine lines, hollowing, dark circles and crow's feet are some of the earliest signs of ageing. Lines of facial expression around the forehead become deeper. And in the lower face, sagging starts to appear and the jawline becomes less defined.

Looking after our skin is a combination of lifestyle, great skincare and carefully chosen procedures, where needed.

In terms of lifestyle, protecting the skin against sunlight is absolutely key. It is estimated that solar radiation is responsible for eighty to ninety per cent of extrinsic ageing of the skin. Other factors involved are air pollution and smoking.

Diet also influences our skin; eat plenty of different coloured fruits and vegetables, oily fish, nuts and seeds. Avoid high intakes of fried food, red meat and sugary foods.

Create a skincare regime that is targeted to your own individual skin type. Listen to your skin and don't overcomplicate your regime. Mornings should be all about protection – sunscreen and a high quality anti-oxidant serum. Your night time routine should be about activation and repair. Vitamin A creams – retinoids – have a multitude of benefits for the skin and are some of the most effective anti-ageing ingredients.

Then take stock of your skin. Are there any specific skin concerns that catch your eye? For certain indications, procedures are the best treatment. For example sun spots respond well to laser and upper face forehead lines respond best to muscle-relaxing injections.

I love the vitamin C serums by Skinceuticals – such as CE Ferulic. These are lightweight serums which help brighten and protect.

Retinoids are an essential part of an anti-ageing regime. I like Flawless Nightly Serum by Dr Sam Bunting, Crystal Retinal by Medik8 or Clinique Smart Night Clinical Retinol.

Sun protection should be broad spectrum to protect against not only UVB, but also UVA, visible light and infra-red. I love the Heliocare range or Anthelios by La Roche Posay.

Rich moisturisers can help protect your skin barrier. Try Triple Lipid Repair by Skinceuticals with ceramides or Cerave PM lotion which contains niacinamide – a multitasking powerhouse of an ingredient.

Before you add any supplements, take stock of your diet. Strip out fried foods, excessive sugars and refined carbohydrates. Ensure you eat plentiful fruits and vegetables and vary this as much as you can. Foods high in essential fatty acids such as oily fish, nuts and seeds can help boost skin health.

In terms of supplements, I always recommend vitamin D, because particularly in the UK it's hard to get all your vitamin D from sunshine, particularly if you seek shade. Omega 3 supplements can be useful, particularly if you don't eat much oily fish. And probiotics are also a very promising area of supplementation."

DR WEDGEWORTH'S TOP SKINCARE TIPS

Sun protection. Without a doubt, the sun is by far and away the greatest cause of extrinsic skin ageing, so protecting your skin from sun damage is one of the most effective ways of slowing the signs of ageing.

Understand your own skin type. We all have different skin types and needs. Identifying your personal needs is key to success so you can use the products that work best for your skin type.

Respect your skin barrier. The outer layer of skin is responsible for holding water in and keeping irritants out. Over-treating your skin with harsh skin care, acid peels and scrubs can damage your skin barrier and sensitise your skin.

Switch up your skincare according to your skin needs. Skin is very dynamic and varies significantly according to your environmental conditions, time of the year and weather. Don't be afraid to listen to your skin and change textures according to how it's reacting.

Don't smoke! Smoking causes premature skin ageing. Tobacco smoke contains high concentrations of toxic chemicals which damage blood vessels and key structural proteins such as collagen.

Consistency. If you want to see changes in your skin, you need to work at it. Active ingredients such as retinoids need to be used daily for at least two to three months before you are likely to see a change, so stick with it!

Simplify. Less is sometimes more in skincare. Create a core routine with cleanser, moisturiser and sunscreen, then add two or three key actives, depending on your individual skin needs. I love ingredients such as retinoids, azelaic acid, niacinamide and vitamin C.

—— Dr Emma Wedgeworth ——

EATING FOR GOOD SKIN

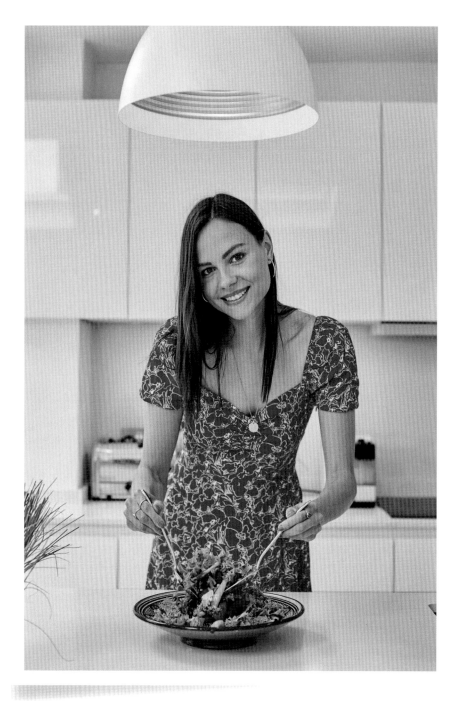

SOPHIE TROTMAN, NUTRITIONIST

One of the themes that keeps emerging throughout this book as you'll find is how important it is to maintain a healthy, balanced diet. Not only will eating well keep your weight where you want it to be, improve your mood and your sleep but what you what you put into your body will show itself in your skin, as Dr Wedgeworth has already touched on. Nutritionist **Sophie Trotman** who has unbelievably gorgeous skin herself, explains how best to eat your way to great skin:

"WITH regards to skin health, what we eat is sorely overlooked. This is astounding, as our cells are created from the food we consume. We quite literally are what we eat! There is little point investing in skincare, only to disregard a nutritious diet. For optimum results, the two need to work in tandem.

Read on to learn about some nutrients we should include in our diets to achieve that smooth, glowing skin we all desire and fight the signs of ageing.

VITAMINS

The beneficial vitamins for skin health include powerful compounds called antioxidants. This has become a marketing buzzword over the past few decades, but do we know what it means and why we should pay attention? Let me break it down for you:

Pollution, sugar, stress, alcohol and certain processed foods increase what's known as 'free radicals' in the body. A build-up of free radicals can lead to oxidative stress and cellular damage which accelerates the skin ageing process.

Antioxidants defend our cells from oxidative stress by neutralising and essentially 'mopping up' the free radicals and slowing down the signs of ageing.

Check out the ORAC score, created by scientists at the National Institute on Ageing that measures the antioxidant capacity of certain foods. Blueberries, spinach, ginger, turmeric and ceremonial-grade matcha are some of the top contenders.

SOPHIE'S TOP VITAMINS FOR SKIN HEALTH

- Vitamin C is a powerful antioxidant that is essential for collagen production. Find it in red pepper, broccoli and oranges.

- Beta-carotene is a nutrient that is converted into vitamin A in the body. High amounts can give the skin a warmer complexion, promoting that enviable natural 'glow'. Sweet potatoes, kale and carrots are great sources of beta-carotene.

- Vitamin E is often deficient in Western diets and levels decrease further as we age. Find it in avocado, salmon, almonds and spinach.

- **Top Tip:** Don't shy away from keeping antioxidant-rich foods in your freezer. Frozen vegetables and fruits are frozen at source, meaning they are often fresher and more nutritious than their fresh counterparts shipped from abroad.

FAT

Over the years, shoddy marketing campaigns and bad science taught us to fear fat. However, we now know that fat is a vital macronutrient that is incredibly beneficial for skin health.

Omega 3 is an essential fat that cannot be made in the body and must be acquired through the diet. Omega 3s are fantastic at helping to seal the skin, maintaining moisture and have anti-inflammatory properties. Try to include two portions of oily fish per week and some omega 3-rich plant foods such as flaxseeds and walnuts. If you don't eat oily fish, a vegan algae-derived supplement may be worth exploring.

Top Tip: Consume a thumb of fat with each meal. This could be seeds, avocado, tahini, extra virgin olive oil or other healthy fats. Avoid trans fats.

PROTEIN

Protein is an essential macronutrient which is often lacking in women's diets. Protein is vital for many functions in the body; essentially it forms the building blocks of tissues and cells. As we age, we tend to require more of this macronutrient.

Animal protein (meat, eggs, dairy and fish) are considered complete proteins, providing all nine essential amino acids. Most plant proteins are known as incomplete proteins; but we can combine certain sources of plant protein to create complete proteins that are beneficial for skin health. There are some plant foods which provide complete proteins like quinoa, soy and buckwheat.

Collagen is the body's most abundant protein and gives our skin elasticity and that much-revered 'plump' look. From our late twenties, collagen levels begin to decrease, leading to signs of ageing like skin sagging and wrinkles. Luckily, we can incorporate sources of collagen in our diet like bone broth and chicken. You could also invest in a collagen supplement, such as the one Anthea takes It is worth noting that vitamin C intake aids collagen synthesis, so even more reason to eat your citrus fruits, berries and leafy green vegetables!

Top Tip: It is necessary to spread our protein intake throughout the day to receive maximum benefit. Try incorporating eggs, fish, yoghurt or nut butter into your breakfasts.

HYDRATION

You've heard it a million times, but water consumption is key! Adequate water consumption means less fine lines, plumper skin, greater elasticity and a brighter complexion. Aim for two litres of water a day and more if you exercise or spend time in the heat.

Top Tip: Herbal non-caffeinated teas contribute towards your water count, but coffee and tea are dehydrating!"

—— **SOPHIE TROTMAN DipION mBANT CNHC** ——
www.sophietrotmannutrition.com
Instagram: @sophietrotmannutrition

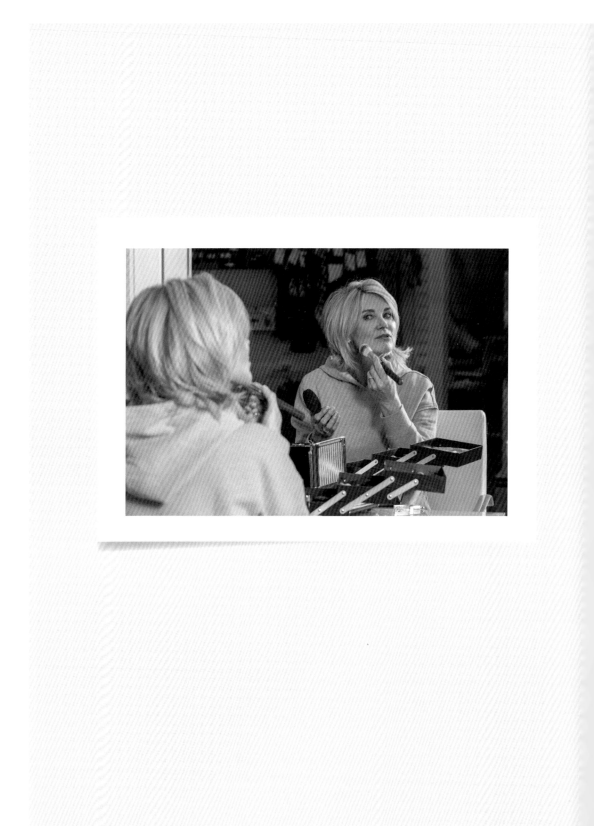

CHAPTER VII

— *Makeup* —

I'VE always had an interest in makeup, bordering on obsession actually. So when I started working in telly and had proper makeup artists showing me how it's done, I was the best pupil ever. The makeup department has always been my happy place, just like the hairdresser's!

Along the way I've learned it's vital to get a really good set of brushes. They're a great investment and should be looked after properly. When my car was broken into, what traumatised me most was having my makeup bag with all my brushes in, stolen. I'd had them for years and was so upset to lose them.

My friend Grace Fodor has a great makeup company called Studio10 and I get some things – not everything – from her. I don't think there's one single company out there from which I'd want to get every product I use and I don't think what you use has to be expensive. It's about trial and error and finding out what works for you.

Over the years there must be very few brands I haven't tried. But as far as my base foundation goes now, I won't use anything other than Bare Minerals powder. I'm not paid to say this. I've never had a free pot of anything in my life from them but for me, Bare Minerals is the go-to. I've used it for years and years and now it's so easy for me to do my makeup, even without a mirror. Sometimes I'll happily make-up my face in the car in ten minutes.

The huge advantage of this particular powder is that it doesn't sit in the crevices of my face and we all have those as we get older. It lasts all day and if I'm going out in the evening, I can just put a bit more on top and buff it up with a brush. I use Bare Minerals Well Rested concealer around my eyes. Like the foundation, it has to be blended in well to get the best results. As you get older, you need to blend better but use less.

Ten years ago, I had a tattoo line over the top of my eyelid, very thin and it shapes my eye. I have it redone every year. And although I've got reasonably thick eyebrows, they're light so I have tattooing within the hair. It doesn't affect the shape; it just makes them look thicker. Eyebrows frame the eyes and are important. To make the best of them, if you want this done, please do your homework because you want them to look as natural as possible. As we age, the heavy overly perfect brow favoured by the young would just look ridiculous on us.

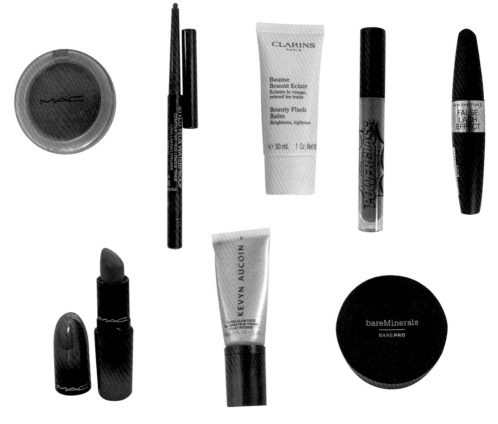

MY MAKEUP ESSENTIALS

With eye shadow I use a palette of natural colours. When I go out I use a little pop of blue or green just to make them stand out. For about twenty years I've used Max Factor mascara which again, I've found works best for me after trying lots of different brands. I have my eyelashes dyed or dye them myself. I use a little caster oil on my lashes and eyebrows at night. It contains fatty acids and vitamin E which are known to encourage hair growth. (I also use this on my hair especially the thin, grey strands around my hair line.)

As I've got older, softer colours work best. Studio10 does a fabulous range of lipsticks which are also blushers.

Kevin Aucoin do lovely highlighters. They give you a dewy bloom which you lose naturally as you get older. I always carry one in my handbag.

A lot of people think I don't wear a lot of makeup but I actually do. It's just that I try and achieve a less-is-more look, more subtle and softer. You have to revisit your look as you get older and tweak and edit over the years.

***

Over the years I've worked with many makeup artists including the wonderful **Helen Hand** from *ITV*. There probably isn't a well-known telly face she hasn't made up at some time or another. She kindly agreed to lend her expertise here so we can all benefit from some professional tips:

"OVER the past twenty-eight years I've been lucky enough to work across all things beauty, hair and makeup, my main job now being a freelance makeup artist. I've worked on loads of different TV shows on numerous channels, photoshoots, red carpet awards, parties, dramas and in the theatre.

How do I choose what I'm going to do or apply when I meet someone? It's easy really. I judge a person's personality and style and go from there. I get to know the person's background, why they're in the studio and coupled with the time of day these things make my choices and decisions for me.

Makeup should be fun and enjoyable for everyone. The nearest I have to rules when it comes to using makeup is great skincare and blend! It can make all the difference between looking good, glam, natural or a mess and having people look at you for all the wrong reasons.

SKINCARE

Skincare is absolutely key to great makeup. Prepping the skin is vital. When you take care of your face you can use less makeup which can contribute to makeup staying on all day, gathering in dry patches or sliding off within the first hour of getting ready. Make sure you always:

Cleanse and tone daily – this is important to cleanse away any traces of dirt, old makeup and pollution from daily life so skin is fresh with no barriers to prevent it being clogged and your moisturiser having to work harder.

Moisturise day and night – the daytime is all about protecting your skin as well as keeping it balanced, hydrated and protected. There are many options to choose from: oil, serum, balm, gel and cream and sometimes you may need to combine two products in order to get the right balance. Always use an SPF to prevent harmful sun damage. Your night time moisturiser is all about restoring, rejuvenating, healing and really treating your skin.

Treat your skin to a weekly treatment – make sure skin is thoroughly cleansed, apply a face exfoliation to stop the build-up of dead skin cells which desquamate every second of the day without us seeing or knowing it's happening. Exfoliation leaves the skin soft and supple so again your mask and moisturiser can do the job they're meant to.

Once you have exfoliated from your decollete up to the forehead, apply a face mask to the same area using the appropriate product for your skin type and needs, leave for fifteen minutes before washing off with a warm flannel. Finish with a cold flannel to awaken and liven the skin.

Apply a tiny amount of eye cream with your smallest fingers so it's light in pressure. The skin in this area is at least forty per cent finer than the rest of your face so you shouldn't use anything too heavy as it can cause puffiness around the eyes. Finish with your moisturiser.

Skin should feel absolutely renewed and makeup can go on to create a smooth, flawless finish. You'll find that you don't need to use a primer under your foundation if you treat your skin with the right products, care on a daily basis and a regular routine.

FOCUS

When looking at what to do, the type of makeup we should wear or what suits us, whether it's the makeup of the season, summertime look going on full glam or uber natural, focus on what you like about yourself and make the most of your best features. Don't focus on what you don't like.

If you love your eyes, make more of them. You can go smoky or natural and add a sexy flicked eye line or none at all. If you have beautifully shaped lips, you can either go bright, natural, dark or full on colour – matte or glossy.

Your biological age really makes no difference at all for me. It depends on you as an individual and the look you want to go for, your personality and style. As you age, all you have to do is make slight adjustments to what you may have applied for the same look when you were younger. Play with colour, texture and really do get to know your face; this is a must. And remember, age is just a number. Full-on smoky eyes can still look stunning as you get older as does a more natural look. Just keep it soft!

As we get older we lose pigment from the places that usually warm our face and keep our look naturally soft which is instantly more youthful to the eye.

Eyebrows and eyelashes fade as well as the hair on our head which can alter a look dramatically as this can change what we see in our skin tone. As well as our skin, hair changes in texture and becomes coarser and often thinner. It's what we can add, take away or mix in texture and tone to keep that youthful glow and prevent us looking outdated, messy and older.

When you wear darker or smoky tones, wash (brush) a colour over the top so the depth doesn't make the eyes look smaller, heavier or flat. Adding a shot of colour like this over the top like a bright pink, red or orange instantly lifts and opens the eye. Make sure eye shadow is blended to soften any hard edges unless that's the look you're going for.

Black is a wonderful shade to use but can sometimes look harsh so mixing it with another colour can add warmth and depth without the hard appearance around the eye area which can be ageing but equally wonderful to enhance your features. Again, just keep it soft.

When it comes to foundation, too much contour and shade can look very sharp, heavy and hard which again is very ageing. Contour and shading should be soft and blended well so the eyes see only a naturally enhanced structure. A good way to check you've picked the right shade with any type of makeup, be it foundation, lipstick, contouring palette or eye shadow is to apply it to the face. Take a small mirror, stand outside and look in natural light to see if it suits.

When eyebrows are a block of colour and too heavy for the face to carry, it can change the structure of how the face and features should look naturally. Keep them as natural looking as possible using an eyebrow pencil to give them colour if they're light or too thin. But avoid that big blocked look.

Too much makeup under the eyes can appear cakey, crepey, wrinkled, saggy and heavy. Try to avoid this by starting your makeup routine with the eyes and forehead first. Cleanse off any makeup that drops (sometimes eye shadow can fall between the lashes resulting in a twenty-four-hour shadow) then continue with the rest of your routine. When you've finished, apply a tiny touch of eye cream, gel or balm then finally your concealer which should go on more smoothly.

***

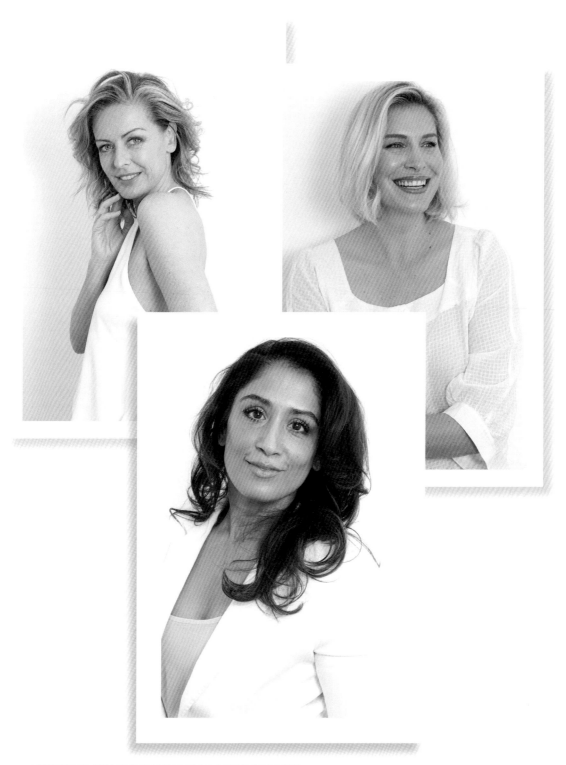

MAKEUP IN ANY DECADE SHOULD LOOK FABULOUS!

LATE TEENS INTO TWENTIES

Remember, you will never have the same naturally youthful skin as you have in your teens and twenties. So avoid camouflaging the face as it's really ageing and you really don't need to. You can conceal anything that needs to be concealed without it looking too heavy. Enjoy your face and the youth you have while you have it!

LATE THIRTIES INTO FIFTIES

For me, this is a cross-over period. These days a lot of women are having their babies later which can be really traumatic on the body and mind. It can increase stress, lack of sleep, eating on the go, worry, hormones all over the place and all of a sudden you have no time for yourself. Coupled with the fact our own parents are getting older where the tables turn and you may have to help them on top of juggling everything else.

It should be the best and calmest time of your life but it's not always that's way. You have to make time for yourself even if it's as little as fifteen to twenty minutes. Exfoliate the body and face, apply a face mask and chill in the bath for fifteen minutes to reboot and feel alive and rejuvenated again. It's a small thing to do but can make all the difference in maintaining the old you.

Menopause can happen at any point but chances increase into your late forties, early fifties. This is where we suffer with lack of oil, hydration, collagen, elasticity in our skin. And we can lose pigment in the areas that keep the warmth in our face.

Tiredness can increase for no reason and not getting enough sleep can really play havoc with the skin so make sure to always have a regular skincare routine and some 'me' time. Don't be frightened to try new products regarding makeup and cosmetics and always seek advice

LATE FIFTIES AND ABOVE

Don't be scared to try new things as we get older. Sometimes we can feel like everything is limited to us. There are no limits or rules as to what you can and can't wear; you just alter or tweak it to suit the newer you that will complement who you are now. Don't forget to love the face you have earned. We can wear the same makeup as we did years before if it's right for our skin type now; colour, products and application just need to be adapted to lift and give the skin a youthful radiant glow without over applying. So there's no such thing as you can't wear the makeup you like as you get older, just make sure the application is smooth and blended well to keep it soft and youthful. Smile often as it helps to lift the face and can instantly take years off you.

I know they say less is more as you get older and I've said it myself but I also say it's an individual thing; sometimes more is better. Your makeup can be strong in colour as long as it's applied and blended well.

Too much of the wrong colour blush or makeup over pigmentation and blemishes can heighten your attention towards it.

Colours such as red or pinkish tones when you have spots or blemishes can draw your attention to them. That goes for all makeup (lipstick, foundation, blush and eyeshadow). This can still happen after you have concealed the problem. If you have applied too much, it can lift easily or the heat from your own skin if not treated correctly can come through or lift the make up throughout the day. This is where skincare comes in to play to see the best results for long lasting make up.

Lipstick can bleed into the skin. To avoid this, when applying your foundation, brush over the lips and blot with powder lightly. Add a lip pencil to seal the lipstick from bleeding and moving. If you find your lipstick disappears easily, add the pencil all over the lips and blot with powder to seal.

Highlighter does what it's called - it highlights - so avoid using it near anywhere you have lines and anything you want to conceal and camouflage. It will exaggerate what you want to cover.

Over powdering the face can look dry and cakey so use a small brush and gently seal the makeup by brush or pat over the areas that overly shine and lifts.

Too much bronzer or tan can take away from your features and give a harder and dry appearance.

When using eyelashes make sure they fit. Cut them down to size and apply the lashes in order to lift the eyes. If the size or length of lashes are too long and heavy for you, they can drag the eyes down which is the opposite to what you want them to do.

Too much metallic eyeshadow can pick up every line and wrinkle so be careful not to overuse this texture.

Throw dry and clogged mascara away. It should go on smoothly and coat all round your lashes without binding the lashes together in clumps.

***

DARK SKIN TONES

Most makeup products today can be used on different skin colours and tones. The darker the skin, the increase of pigmentation can occur due to having more melanin cells in the skin.

Skin can be darker around the mouth, chin and eyes. We all have many different tones within our skin colour so to achieve a flawless finish, add a red, yellow or orange base to your foundation or blend two or more foundations. Concealer needs a lot of red or orange pigment to lift the skin as anything too light can appear flat and ashen looking.

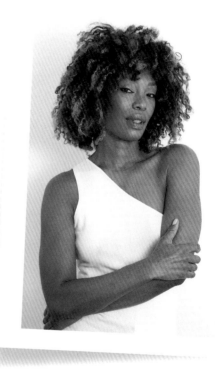

Dark skin tones call for richer, warmer colours when it comes to makeup. They can take bolder tones such as gold, berries and even oranges.

Some of my favourite brands which I use on darker skin, include:

Charlotte Tilbury Airbrush Lawless 14 cool - this foundation has great coverage leaving the skin looking radiant and even. It applies really well and evens out skin tones without looking heavy and cakey.

Concealer Charlotte Tilbury Magic away in number 13 - this is light and covers well without looking crepey.

Pat McGrath Labs, Fenty Beauty, Iman, Cover FX and Nars all have a wide range of shades and colours to suit all skins. Bobbi Brown and Mac cosmetics have a brilliant range which can be adaptable to mix and achieve that perfect skin tone."

—— **Helen Hand** ——

MAKEUP FOR MATURE SKIN MADE EASY

I've already mentioned Grace Fodor. She founded the incredibly successful makeup brand Studio10 in 2016, especially for the mature woman. (Grace herself is a young fifty-six!)

She's absolutely the perfect person to offer advice here: her passion is to help women age well with makeup and so her brand is most definitely Pro-Age rather than Anti-Ageing.

This is what Grace has to say on the subject:

"LOOKING good on the outside can give us the boost we need to feel good on the inside, and makeup is a great tool for giving us this sense of confidence. The good news is, applying makeup doesn't have to be time-consuming or confusing. This four-step routine – prime, perfect, shade and shape – will fit seamlessly into your morning regime, to give you flawless skin and lit-from-within radiance, no matter what your age.

Before putting on anything else, apply sunscreen under your makeup. Even on a grey day, the sun's harmful UV rays can damage your skin, leaving you vulnerable to developing sun-related problems such as pigmentation, premature ageing, wrinkles and even skin cancers. Recent studies have shown that sunscreen also helps to reverse the common signs of ageing, such as wrinkles and hyperpigmentation.

I recommend Heliocare Oil-Free Gel SPF50. This is an ultra-light formula that melts into the skin with a dry-touch, matte finish. It's suitable for all skin types, including oily and combination complexions.

1. PRIME

As we get older, collagen and elastin production start to slow down, resulting in wrinkles, and the sebaceous glands produce less oil, meaning our skin can become dry.

The trick here is to use a primer on the skin after you've moisturised and before you apply foundation, to create an even base for makeup and to keep products from settling into any fine lines. A good primer will not only smooth the complexion, but also add radiance. I recommend looking for one with gold rather than silvery tones, as this will look more natural on the skin.

Our Youth Lift Glow-plexion is an all-in-one fool-proof product, enriched with a special blend of hyaluronic acid that helps to lock in moisture and hydrate the skin.

Its smooth, creamy and glitter-free formula instantly minimises pores and evens out the complexion. You can use it under your makeup, but it can also be mixed with foundation or a tinted moisturiser, used on top of makeup as a highlighter, or mixed with body lotion for an all-over glow.

If you suffer from enlarged pores, try Smashbox's Photo Finish Pore Minimizing Primer. Its oil-free formula dramatically reduces the look of pores while smoothing and prepping skin for flawless makeup application.

2. PERFECT

Over the years, our skin goes through a lot. Years of sun exposure may lead to age spots, redness, blemishes and pigmentation issues. Once you've primed your skin, it's time to cover up any pigmentation you may have. I recommend a medium-to-full coverage foundation with hydrating properties to nourish the skin throughout the day.

Our Age Repair Perfect Canvas SPF30 Foundation evens out your skin tone without looking cakey, meaning there's no need for concealer. The colour-adjusting formula reflects the light for a bright, dewy-looking effect, while optical diffusing pigments blend and buff seamlessly, giving a real-skin finish.

3. SHADE

With ageing, the outer skin layer (epidermis) thins and the number of pigment-containing cells (melanocytes) decreases, meaning our skin can look sallow and pale.

For an instant complexion pick-me-up, I recommend adding a flush of healthy colour and glow using a peach-toned blush. It's best to avoid powder blushers on mature skin, as they can dehydrate your complexion and can collect in fine lines. A liquid blush is a better option, as it doesn't sit on top of the skin, and can be easily blended and buffed for a smooth finish.

Try our bestselling Plumping Blush Glow-plexion. It's universally flattering, with orange pigments to add warmth to your skin, and pearl highlights to brighten the complexion.

4. SHAPE

As we age our skin loses collagen and elasticin, the glue that helps the body maintain its shape and structure by binding tissues and cells. Think of this as Spanx for the face. Adding shape and definition while enhancing features and creating a natural looking lift.

Contouring is a quick and easy way to sculpt and define your facial features, adding dimension to your face. The principle is to use makeup that is slightly darker or lighter than your actual skin colour to create natural contours. Light shades (highlighter) will bring features forward while darker shades (contouring products or a darker toned foundation) will make them recede.

Our Radiance Glow Bronzing Veil is my secret for a natural healthy colour and the perfect summer tan. The subtle red-brown tones instantly enhance your complexion, revealing natural warmth and healthy skin-true colour while the matte consistency makes the powder perfect for contouring and creating the illusion of a depth and shadow.

To apply, take the darker shade on an angled cheek brush and trace the product along the hollows of your cheeks in a "3" shape that follows your hairline, under cheekbone and jawline. Next, for multi-dimensional radiance, bring the light back into your face by applying the illuminating powder to the areas that reflect light naturally: your forehead, the bridge of your nose and the top of your cheekbones.

Once you've finished defining your face, it's time to add shape to the brows and lips.

Brows can become thinner as we age. Combat this with brow-defining products to open up your eyes and frame your face. I recommend our Brow Lift Perfecting Brow Pencil. It's long-wearing and buildable, and its unique ash-tone mimics hair and adjusts for a true-to-you finish. Apply using short, hair-like strokes in an upward motion for shapely brows that help lift and enhance your eyes. Once finished, take the skin-toned highlighter and apply underneath your brow bone to highlight and lift the eyes.

Then, to create balance between the top and bottom halves of your face, it's important to line the lips. As we age, our lips lose their full shape as the fat pads underneath the skin begin to break down. To create a plumper lip, overline slightly with a your-lips-but-better liner, topped with a gloss, to add shine and definition. Try our Age Reverse Perfecting Lipliner using the rose shade just outside the lip line, and the cream shade to highlight and line the cupid's bow to accentuate the lips further.

STUDIO I **10**

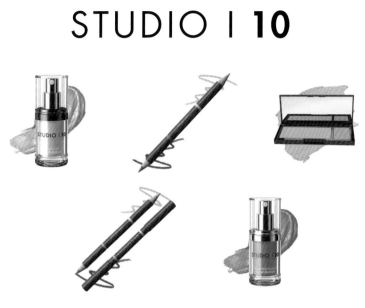

WWW.STUDIO10BEAUTY.COM

MENOPAUSE MAKEUP

Hormonal shifts during menopause can cause several changes to the skin, resulting in breakouts, redness and dullness. Rosacea can be triggered, so combat this by applying a light wash of a green colour corrector to tone down any redness on your skin. Our Age Defy Skin Perfector palette includes a feather-light, green-toned concealer packed with antioxidant-rich, strengthening and firming active ingredients.

Hot flushes and excessive sweating can create havoc with a beautifully made-up face, so I recommend applying your makeup using our Double Ended Face Brush to avoid transferring the oil from your fingers to your face and to keep your temperature down, which is especially important if you're having a hot flush.

Waterproof makeup and long-lasting formulas will also be your best friends during this time! Our Liquid Foil I-Radiance and double-ended I-Lift Longwear Liner will make the perfect additions to your routine. The multi-purpose, budge-proof and waterproof formulas highlight, shape, define and enhance the eyes while ensuring no smudging or caking when you're feeling the heat.

Blotting papers are a must for absorbing any excess oil and keeping your makeup in place. Shiseido Oil-Control Blotting Papers are easy to keep in your handbag to freshen up your makeup on the go.

I also recommend keeping a cooling spray in your bag to freshen your skin and keep it hydrated throughout the day.

I love MegsMenopause Rosey Rain Facial Cooling Spray – it's infused with natural rose and marshmallow root extracts to relieve irritation and help soothe and calm the skin.

Experiencing the menopause doesn't mean you have to stop wearing the makeup you love. Ultimately, any colours, formulas and products that make you feel confident and the best version of yourself are going to be the right ones for you, regardless of your age – but there's always room to make some simple adjustments to switch up your makeup routine and make the most of your mature skin."

—— **Grace Fodor** ——

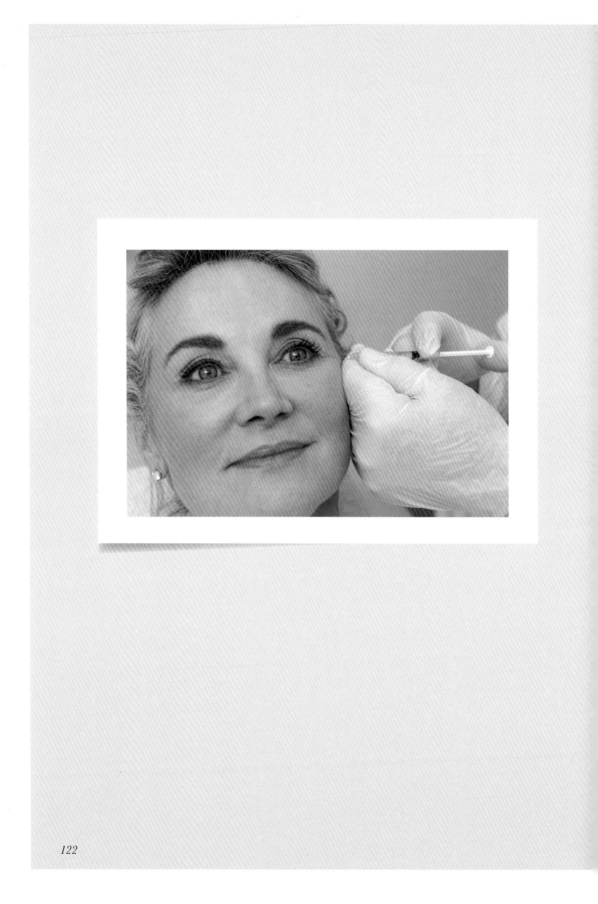

CHAPTER VIII

—— Nip and Tuck ——

MY thoughts on this one are completely open and non-judgmental and as you would expect I love the phrase, 'Tidy up as you go along'. I firmly believe that as long as you don't become addicted to surgery, there's nothing wrong with a bit of nip and tuck if it makes you feel good about yourself. Why not?

But the good news is, before you get anywhere near a knife there is so much you can achieve to stem the onset of ageing through non-invasive treatments. To be honest I've always been a little bemused by people saving up for a face lift as if it's the holy grail of youth when they plainly haven't looked after their body, teeth, skin or hair which are all pretty easy and cheap to take care of by comparison.

A good overall appearance is what you're trying to achieve so it's crucial your face and body look like they belong to the same person. I've seen so many women with tight faces and bodies that look like someone else's.

Before you start researching surgeons, there are a number of non-invasive treatments out there you could try first if you want a little extra help to achieve the look you want. I'm not suggesting these are right for every woman – and I certainly am not encouraging women to fork out for procedures which I know can be expensive and for some, a step too far. I'm only describing what I've had done myself at times and have been happy with. We're all different.

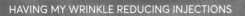

SINGLE-USE ONLY

HAVING MY WRINKLE REDUCING INJECTIONS

I've seen great results with wrinkle reducing injections, fillers and Profhilo to help restore shape and form to the face, IPL to remove uneven pigmentation, Invisalign and whitening to straighten and brighten up teeth, a good haircut and colour to make the most of the hair. It also helps to lose those extra pounds with a good diet and exercise to tone up and only resort to surgery as a last ditch option – if you absolutely have to! And again, even with surgery, you'll have no judgement from me. It's all about what works for you and what will make you feel good about yourself.

I've kept on top of all of the above but what I couldn't fix without surgery, were my small, saggy little tits or as a friend called hers, 'An egg in a sock'. Another friend referred to hers as 'Spaniels' ears' and then there's my friend whose reduction literally changed her life who thought of her boobs as her 'Bloody boulders.'

To be honest I think boob jobs, as they are commonly called, are as normal now as getting your teeth capped, and most people I know can't wait to share their procedure with their friends. At one 'unveiling' party I went to, Grace arrived looking amazing, glowing with confidence, wearing a dress she'd never have bought before because she couldn't have rocked it in the same way (yes it was backless).

Thousands of boob jobs are performed in the UK each year, mainly enlargements. However, if you want one, please do your homework and choose wisely whose hands you are going to put your assets into.

If you've ever watched the TV programme *Botched* you'll know how terribly wrong it can all go and you wonder how those cowboy surgeons get away with it. Personally, I can't praise my surgeon enough. Pinky and Perky look natural, not too big, not too small. They have balanced out my body shape, ie the circumference of my boobs and bum more or less match and although when I first had them done I looked in horror at these strange new accessories, I now love them.

I once sat next to a plastic surgeon at a dinner and he told me, the key to a successful surgery is when your friends don't notice and they just say, 'You look well, have you been on holiday?' Yes, and I had the breast time!

— *A* —

I've been seeing Dr Andrew Weber at Bodyvie Medi-Clinic in Richmond-Upon-Thames for many of my medical, aesthetic and skincare needs for about twenty years and can't recommend him highly enough. I am not on his payroll and I would never endorse anyone I did not have full confidence in.

Those of you who follow me on Instagram, know I've always been transparent about the various treatments I use and I am always happy to try new ones. As always, I'll leave it to the expert to explain what procedures I opt for and what they do:

"ANTHEA combines line and wrinkle injections, fillers and Profhilo with therapies such as lasers, facials and micro-needling treatments, which help work on long-term maintenance and improvement of skin quality.

Line and Wrinkle Reducing Injections – Treatment involves the administration of a botulinum toxin into specific facial muscles via tiny injections. The botulinum toxin binds onto nerve endings, blocking receptors and stopping the release of a transmitter which stimulates muscles into contractions. In short, it can soften, reduce, or completely stop the formation of active lines, which over time develop into passive lines (ones that are always there!). Treatments are tailored to patients' desired outcome and we always work to achieve natural looking results, avoiding that 'wind-tunnel effect' you see so often from over administration.

My ethos has always been 'less is more' and trying to 'maintain a healthy and natural look without altering appearances'. I believe that many aesthetic treatments offer a great insurance policy for the skin. By softening and slowing line formation and maintaining skin health, the ageing process can be slowed down, reducing the requirements for more invasive treatments down the line.

Fillers – We do not use permanent fillers at our clinic, as management of these products is far more complicated. We favour hyaluronic acid-based fillers, as we have an enzyme to dissolve the product if necessary, or should patients decide they do not like the aesthetic result.

We offer a range of leading filler brands which produce natural looking results to restore lost volume, fill lines, target dark eyes and under-eye circles, hydrate skin and restore a youthful appearance. Results are dependent on the product but typically last twelve months.

Profhilo – This is unique in that it is a super hydrator, which works at improving skin quality, including collagen and elastin production, as well as dermal thickness and hydration.

Profhilo is favoured for the slow, natural and gradual improvement that it offers patients. Results are cumulative following two to three sessions. Patients love that it makes them look 'rested and healthy', rather than altered in appearance. It's the type of treatment that leaves other people thinking how well you look, rather than them assuming you have had a cosmetic alteration. Profhilo really has been a revolutionary treatment within our industry! It is an absolute game changer for providing patients with a solution for skin quality improvement.

From our twenties we begin to lose collagen at a rate of about one per cent per year. After the menopause this increases to about six per cent per year. With this in mind, I try to emphasise to patients the importance of not only receiving the treatments which provide an instant hit, such as dermal fillers. But to ensure that treatments such as Profhilo are administered alongside, to ensure that we are addressing skin quality.

The most common procedure in clinic is still line and wrinkle reducing injections, but Profhilo has worked its way into second place. Patients like it because it's natural. It lasts longer and results are cumulative, they are over a period of time. It's not as if you leave home with small lips and you return with whopping great big ones because you've had a filler put in. This is much more subtle which every woman wants.

INTIMATE HEALTH

The majority of our patients are female and predominantly aged between thirty five and sixty-five. All these women have one thing in common: they will all go through the menopause. It's the effects of that that we try to discuss quite openly. We discuss HRT of which we're strong advocates, the effect of the menopause on the skin and what to expect. The perimenopause can start about ten years before the menopause so symptoms can start quite early.

There are parts of the body that are oestrogen-sensitive, including vaginal tissue. So many women are going to get vaginal atrophy, stress incontinence, dryness, pain, recurrent urinary tract infections and so on.

As well as HRT we offer treatments like laser and PRP for vaginal symptoms. The laser treatment will stimulate the production of collagen and elastin to help increase natural lubrication and comfort. It will help with stress incontinence. We can combine that with PRP which involves taking blood from the patient and injecting it into the anterior vaginal wall. It will thicken the mucosa by stimulating the production of more collagen which gives a bulking effect and better support for the bladder and the urethra. The results are very positive."

—— **Dr Andrew Weber** ——

We all know by now that as we get older, our faces change. We only have to look in a mirror to notice the odd sun spot or wrinkle or the slightly sagging jowls. **Fiona Sellars** who is Director and Lead Clinician at Surrey Hills Skin Clinic explains what's happening behind these changes during the ageing process:

"GENETICS, lifestyle and ethnicity play a big part in how we age. Ageing can manifest in many ways. Generally men tend to notice thinning of hair, skin may have a look of tiredness or stress and take on a grey pallor. Women tend to be more prone to fine lines, pigmentation changes and an overall loss of skin firmness and lack of fullness.

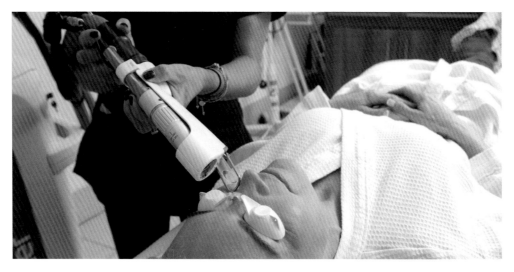

HAVING LASER TREATMENT AT BODYVIE MEDI-CLINIC IN RICHMOND-UPON-THAMES

Women begin to experience and notice changes to their faces around the perimenopausal/menopausal years. Again, our genetics, health, lifestyle and ethnicity play a big part. Patients who have enjoyed tanning and have a history of regular use of sunbeds in their twenties, will often notice fine lines and pigment changes earlier due to premature ageing from ultraviolet light. Other lifestyle factors of course include habits such as smoking and alcohol intake.

WHEN DOES IT ALL START TO CHANGE?

Typically, our faces start to change during our thirties but if we're lucky, not until our forties! We lose volume and this, coupled with changes to our bone composition can result in weaker underlying structures causing a heavy look to our face. This heaviness can lead to looking permanently tired and very commonly a saggy appearance to the lower face and in particular to the jowl area. Interestingly, women are often subconsciously aware of these changes and compensate by wearing hair up high, or styling hair into a short bob to rebalance this look of heaviness.

Overall general health can play a part in how we age. For example, if I review a patient with diabetes, as part of the consultation I ask how regulated their blood insulin is. If levels are erratic and therefore poorly controlled for a prolonged period of time, skin can become dry, have less collagen and less blood supply. As a result, this can cause the skin to appear aged.

There is no doubt about it, genetics play a huge part in how we age. I am by no means an expert in dentistry but how the jaw and teeth are positioned in a patient, can determine how they age to the lower face. It is often a familial trait and defined by a dentist as an overbite or overjet. From an aesthetic perspective, these patients have a 'weak chin' leading to changes in the jowl and neck area often from the early thirties. If the jaw and dentition are left uncorrected there is a certain amount that can be achieved with dermal fillers. However, in my opinion, correcting the underlying structure would be preferable.

It is not uncommon for me to review patients in their mid to late twenties conscious of a frown line typically in between their brows that remains when their face is rested. In these younger patients, I tend to ask if they notice this same trait in either one of their parents and ninety-nine point nine per cent of the time the answer is YES! It's debatable as to whether this is a learnt behaviour from early years or indeed a genetic predisposition. As much as I am an advocate of not starting injectable treatments young, patients such as this have a clear indication and are conscious. I actively treat this younger cohort of patients as the line left untreated will undoubtedly deepen and create a 'cross' look when their face is rested. If they have presented to the clinic with concerns at a young age this will not change as they get older, just as the line gets deeper it will be more complicated to treat.

CAN WE AGE GRACEFULLY?

YES! The key to ageing gracefully is to look after our body, mind and soul and it's as simple as that! Facial aesthetic treatments such as dermal fillers and wrinkle relaxation treatments can be used sympathetically to reduce the negative attributes associated with ageing. For example, the look of tiredness, sagginess, anger or sadness can be an emotion that is etched on a face when at rest. This can affect self-esteem and confidence so when these emotions are effectively treated in the clinic, I'm not only treating the face, I'm treating the mind and soul too.

FIONA'S TOP FIVE AESTHETIC TREATMENTS

- Dermal fillers
- Wrinkle relaxation injections
- Injectable skin boosters/ hydration eg Profhilo
- Microneedling
- Radiofrequency skin tightening

FIONA'S HACKS

- The earlier you look after your skin the better. If you do this from your twenties onwards, your skin will repay you later in life
- Wear SPF 45 or above all year round. Although UVB becomes stronger during the spring and summer months, UVA stays consistent all year round. These UVB rays penetrate deeper and ages us
- Take Vitamin D during the winter months
- Moisturiser is your best friend, find one that works for you, and hydrate with water!

I wholeheartedly feel ageing is a mind-set! Learn to be comfortable in your skin, be confident, use your smile and don't be afraid to embrace the age you are regardless of whether you seek aesthetic treatments or not.

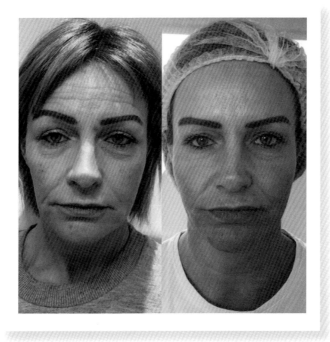

BEFORE AND AFTER DERMAL FILLERS AND WRINKLE RELAXING INJECTIONS

Aesthetic treatments are very personal and are by no means a fit for all. However, if you are conscious of the signs of ageing and have been sitting on the fence about 'tweakments', book a consultation to allow some fact-finding.

Recommendations are always a good start and ensure the practitioner you are seeing is a regulated healthcare professional. Expect to pay a consultation fee as this reflects both knowledge and experience. The doctor, nurse or dentist can assess your concerns, discuss options and manage expectations accordingly. Aesthetic treatments are a journey, treatment plans often change and evolve and the ideal is to have a practitioner you trust, that will be honest and share your journey with you.

The art is to create the look of extreme wellness. Not puffy and certainly not treated in any way!"

—— **Fiona Sellars** ——

PERFECT YOUR SMILE

One of the first things you notice when you meet someone is their teeth. You can tell whether a person has neglected their smile or taken good care of their teeth and I definitely do.

I have regular dental check-ups, brush twice a day using an electric toothbrush and I floss. It was instilled in me as a child that I could never go to bed without cleaning my teeth and I never do – even if I'm inebriated. I also get my teeth whitened on a regular basis.

You're lucky if you've never had to have braces but unfortunately, many people aren't blessed with straight, perfect looking teeth. It can be ageing, particularly as our teeth move all the time and it can affect your confidence.

If you missed out on braces as a teenager and still aren't happy with your smile, it's never too late to do something about it, especially with all the new procedures and techniques which certainly weren't around when I was growing up.

Dr Kunal Patel runs the hugely successful, super hi-tech, fully digitalised Love Teeth Dental clinic in Cheam which was the first clinic in the UK to achieve Invisalign Diamond accreditation within a year. (You might have seen him pop up on TV during the first lockdown as he and his team helped out with the Nightingale Hospital in London and donated thousands of pieces of PPE to the NHS.)

Considered one of the rising young lights in dentistry in the UK, Dr Patel is passionate about achieving that all-important healthy smile and is particularly talented when it comes to the use of Invisalign which has literally transformed the way teeth are straightened without the need for unsightly braces. Obviously, this isn't a cheap option but if you've always been self-conscious about your smile, especially as you've got older, it's definitely worth investigating. As Dr Patel explains, our teeth are always on the move and it sometimes reaches the point where action is needed.

"THROUGHOUT our entire life, our teeth never stop moving. They are attached to our bone with tiny ligaments which act like springs, giving us the perception of pressure. This is also how we are able to move teeth into desired positions using orthodontic methods. As we get older our bone levels can reduce therefore giving us less support and this can cause teeth to move into undesired positions more easily.

Teeth movement and general 'wear and tear' as we grow older, can make it more difficult to eat as tooth surface wears and if we lose teeth it can affect the shape of our face also. It's common to experience tooth loss due to bone loss causing teeth to become loose and need extraction.

Old fillings and dental crowns become loose or wear away requiring replacements. Bruxism (teeth grinding) affects approximately ten per cent of the population and goes untreated by many; this eventually leads to teeth fractures or loss also.

Many people are terrified of the dentist – find one whom you can trust and will put you at ease – and choose to leave their dental problems untreated. This is totally the wrong way to go. Teeth loss can result in having to have more severe dental treatments down the road such as dental implants or dentures. Or it can lead to teeth fracture resulting in possible dental crowns. These are all costly and time consuming treatments which could easily be avoided with early action.

THE BEST WAYS TO CARE FOR OUR TEETH

• Preventative action is the best way

• Make regular dental hygiene and dental examination visits. Every three to twelve months is sensible, depending on the condition of your teeth

• Use a regular and effective oral hygiene routine. This should include brushing teeth twice daily and flossing daily

• Avoid sugary food and drinks as much as possible. Try drinking through a straw if you can't beat a sugar craving

• Avoid snacking and have 'naughty' treats only during meal times

• No rinsing after brushing, so toothpaste remains on teeth

WHAT IS INVISALIGN?

Invisalign is the most advanced, reliable and efficient aligner system in the world in my opinion and involves wearing aligners - clear braces - for between seven weeks and six months, depending on the severity of the case. (Sometimes it takes even longer.)

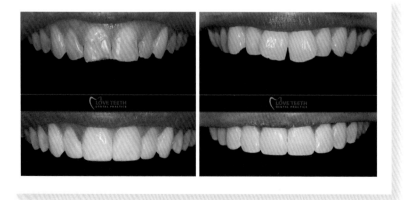

BEFORE AND AFTER INVISALIGN

It is a discreet way to straighten your teeth predicatably. As aligners are removable, it is easy to brush teeth to keep teeth and gums healthy.

Straight and aligned teeth will help make sure you bite correctly causing less tooth wear and risk of teeth fracture and/or loss. And straighter teeth are easier to clean, helping them stay brighter and whiter.

Obviously there's a cost implication and if Invisalign is not for you, the best solution is to maintain a healthy, balanced diet with a good oral hygiene routine. Do not wait for a problem to arise. Think of your teeth as a car requiring an MOT and regular servicing in order to prevent costly bills later on."

—— **Dr Kunal Patel** ——

THE EYES HAVE IT

I finally plucked up the courage to get laser corrective surgery on my eyes fairly recently, after months of preparation by my excellent – and very patient – ophthalmic surgeon, **Mr Ali Mearza** of OCL Vision. I was fed-up of forever looking for my glasses and it's something I'd been desperate to have done for years and years. So I thought, let's go for it.

Not everyone needs laser surgery or wants it and would rather spend their hard-earned cash on something else entirely! But what we all need is good eye health; Mr Mearza kindly agreed to give me his expert tips to share with you on how we can best take care of our precious assets as we get older:

"JUST like the rest of our bodies, our eyes undergo an ageing process. The main thing that occurs is the loss of focussing ability of the lens within the eyes which becomes apparent in the mid-forties onwards. We have to hold things further away to read and then have to succumb to reading glasses when our arms aren't long enough. The power of the reading glasses then needs to increase as we age as the lens in our eyes stiffen further and we lose more focussing power.

From the mid-sixties onwards, cataracts can start developing which is essentially the natural lens becoming cloudy over time. This can occur earlier or later than the mid-sixties but eventually reaches a stage where it affects vision and intervention is required to restore vision. The loss of reading vision can be corrected by either laser vision correction or by lens surgery depending on findings at examination. Cataracts, although one of life's inevitabilities, can be treated with cataract surgery and appropriate lens replacement depending on the needs of the individual.

Other things that occur with age are reduced tear production which can result in dry eyes and irritation as well as fluctuating vision. Changes to the retina can also occur as we age giving rise to problems such as macular degeneration which in turn can affect the vision. Growths and changes to the top layer of the eye as well as the eyelids can also occur depending on genetic predisposition and the amount of sun exposure sustained over time.

How can we protect our eyes against ageing? There's not much we can do to counteract the loss of focussing power of the lens but having a healthy active lifestyle with a well-balanced diet can go some way to delaying or at least helping with some of the eye-related changes that occur with age. Smoking for example is a big no no. It can accelerate cataract formation and has a well-recognised association with age-related macular degeneration. Wearing sunglasses in sunny conditions is also important in avoiding any sun-related damage to the eyes which can accumulate over time.

Are there foods/supplements that can help? A well-balanced diet and plenty of water intake is important for eye health. There are specific supplements available to prevent macular degeneration and for overall eye health and these are available at most good chemists and health food shops. However, a balanced diet with lots of greens will often achieve the same thing. Our blog post, *'Top super foods for healthy eyes'* has some more information. Go to www.oclvision.com/blog/superfoods-for-healthy-eyes."

—— **Mr Ali Mearza** ——

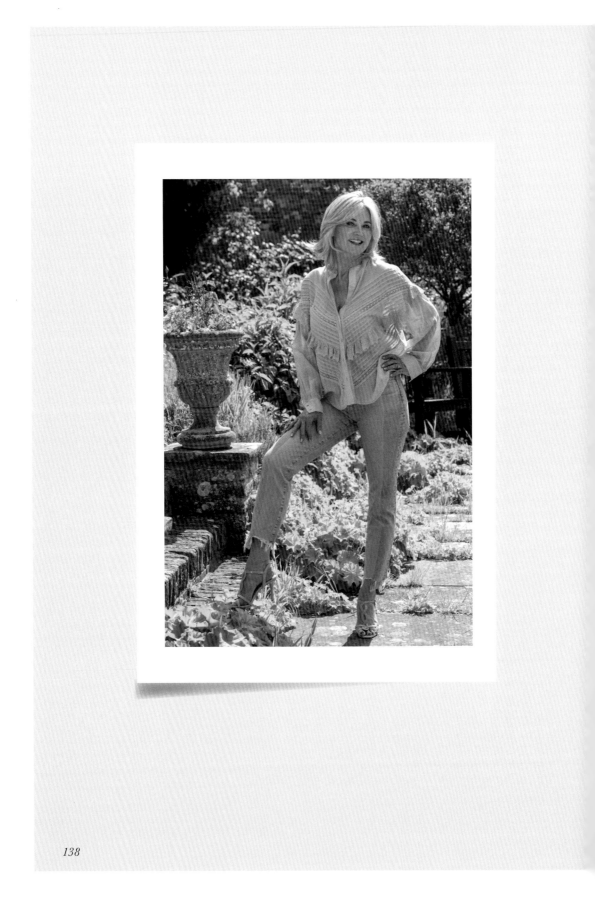

CHAPTER IX

— Style —

We all have 'style'; it's subjective, it's ours, we own it but as we age our look has to be tweaked, edited and freshened up. Often what we rock when we're young just looks an ageing mess on an older person, as though you dressed in the dark from the ironing basket or in the words of my mother Jean who I've never seen in a pair of leggings, 'Mutton dressed as lamb'. If you're not bothered, then you're probably not reading this book, so we'll get on with it and not sit on the fence!

I've had many turfings out over the years but the one I remember with clarity was when my stepdaughter Claudia took over. We were living together. She'd seen me at my worst and needed me back to my old self, firing on all cylinders. At the time she was going through her, 'everything's been through a mixed wash, rammed in the tumble dryer and stayed there for a few days' stage, so I was right to be dubious of her assistance. But my husband had recently left me for a twenty-four year-old so with my confidence at a big fat zero, I was wide open to help.

As Claudia channelled her 'inner Trinny', the reject pile got higher. I was in panic mode saying goodbye to old favourites, and clothes that had memories of another life sewn into in every seam. Was she right? Mostly, although in the dead of night I did extract from the bag, pieces from my trusty cowgirl look; items that turned me into a sad *Bananarama* groupie, probably last worn on *GMTV* or under the heading 'No longer age appropriate' stayed exactly where they were.

THIS DRESS IS FROM FEATHER & STITCH - SUPPORTING INDEPENDENT BOUTIQUES

I have over the years been lucky enough to work with some wonderful stylists, and had the opportunity to 'play' in their dressing up box of clothes bought to shoots. I adore clothes and professionally learnt many years ago I work in a visual medium and fifty per cent of the gig is looking the part.

My greatest lesson however was moving from *Blue Peter* to *GMTV*, let me tell you, for the nineties, that was a fashion leap! What I hadn't informed my employers when they took me on was I had enough 'smart clothes' to get me from Monday's show to Thursday's. After that I was in trouble. So, on the Friday morning when I sat next to the smartly-suited Eamonn Holmes wearing a chunky jumper, flirty pleated black skirt and over the knee socks, the shock was too much and I was marched off very quickly with the Wardrobe Mistress and instructions to 'smarten the girl up and get her a nice sleek bob or something.'

Clothes can give you confidence and yes under the sentimental heading I still have the pink suit I wore the day I found mine. It will stay in my wardrobe forever, standing as a reminder of that scared inner soul that eventually looked down the lens and said quietly to herself, 'I've got this.' Within a year, together with Nicky Clarke's magic scissors (we resisted the sleek bob, my curly hair won't do it), I'd won 'Best Dressed Woman in Television'. You have no idea just how much that award which sits on my dressing table meant to me.

PS - My wardrobe has obviously improved because Claudia has recently been known to utter the unthinkable 'Can I borrow?' Or maybe she's just getting older?

PPS - I do wear leggings and officially wear workout gear even when I have no intention of working out, but for some strange reason makes me move around better (see Alexander Technique).

PPPS - I still dream about that rara skirt I wore over white bell bottoms and with a tiny white Ralph Lauren jumper. But may I add, in my defense of flares, they're back (did they ever go away?) and if you want to make our bum look good, flares and heels says the Jean Queen herself, Donna Ida. I have Donna's jeans in black, white and denim. 'Wow' said my friend Alison, this book's photographer when she saw me in them. 'They do your bum a favour.'

— *A* —

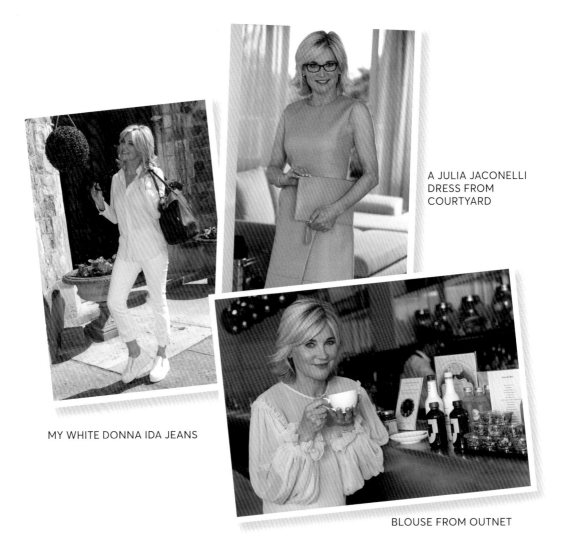

A JULIA JACONELLI DRESS FROM COURTYARD

MY WHITE DONNA IDA JEANS

BLOUSE FROM OUTNET

I adore clothes and love nothing more than shopping for an event or special occasion. Sometimes I have the help of a stylist if I have a work-related function to go to and need to know I won't rock up wearing the same outfit as the host! Other times, I enjoy mooching about in small boutiques. I think it's really important to support independent stores and I have a few firm favourites I've shopped at over the years.

One boutique in particular is Courtyard in Guildford which is owned by my now very good friend **Julia Jaconelli** who has 'dressed' me for about seventeen years. It won Best Independent Womenswear stores in the UK a few years ago and Julia keeps it stocked up with sustainable collections of everything from belts to occasion dresses.

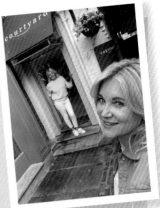

"ANTHEA has been a loyal customer of mine for many years and has been a great ambassador for Courtyard which has been lovely. It's such a pleasure seeing her looking great in the outfits she chooses.

During the years she has been a customer we have agreed that while it's important to stay fashionable and stylish we need to be aware of the limitations of certain things we can and cannot wear. It's important to cover up the parts of our body we don't want to draw attention to that might not be quite the same as they were when we were younger but also great to accentuate the good bits !

I like to buy collections that are sustainable in that they will last for more than one season both in quality and in style . Also clothes that are produced ethically, that are easy to wear and that appeal to a wide age range.

Being an independent store I think it's important to provide newness and freshness each season. I love the challenge of finding new brands that can't be found in other stores in the UK. However I also stick with brands that are well established and that have been popular with our clients for many years.

All occasions are provided for so we stock knitwear, jeans , casual wear , holiday wear , special occasion wear and of course accessories including bags, shoes, scarves , belts and jewellery . Our customers love the fact that this is a one stop shop where they can find everything they need. I feel that independent boutiques are becoming more and more popular as they offer such an individual service and have a uniqueness not provided by the larger chains. It's so great that we have such a loyal clientele which continues to grow each season as more people discover us".

—— **Julia Jaconelli** ——
www.courtyarduk.co.uk

One tip I'd like to share before passing you on to a professional, is trawl magazines and Instagram for a look that catches your eye. Before whipping out the credit card, check your own wardrobe. So many of us have the items already but we just haven't arranged them in the right order.

Now let me introduce you to stylist **Arabella Boyce** who has helped me out many a time. She's also dressed some of the biggest names in showbiz such as Dame Joan Collins, Liv Tyler and David Beckham:

"WHEN I was first asked to write a style piece for Anthea's book I was delighted to help. Anthea is funny, irreverent, quirky and in some ways an icon of the nineties, epitomising the perfectly coiffed TV bombshell, the pneumatic blonde in bold pop colours, neat neon skirt suits and a nod to Versace. She was never grunge but always naughty, albeit with her well-kempt and neat appearance every day on our screens, a look which is copied over and over again today as seen at Balmain and Balenciaga.

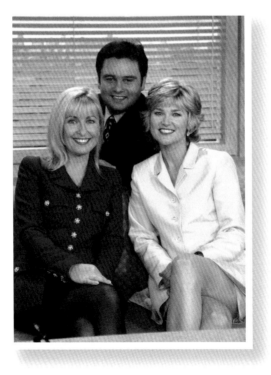

ANTHEA ROCKING HER NINTIES NEON TELLY SUIT AT *GMTV* WITH FIONA PHILLIPS AND EAMONN HOLMES

I've worked with Anthea for over fifteen years. She has great humour, noting my appearance at Sainsbury's one day, that I didn't look as glamorous as I did in my pictures from a wedding in South Africa where the theme of the party was 'Glamouflage'.

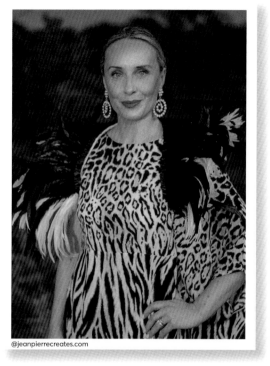

@jeanpierrecreates.com

'YOU DIDN'T LOOK LIKE THAT WHEN I SAW YOU IN SAINSBURY'S LAST WEEK!'

This perfectly encapsulates our relationship. The idea of clothes being transformative. The idea that clothes can empower you and make you feel fabulous and happy.

I've worked for twenty-four years in an industry where my job is to inspire and make people feel amazing about themselves through their clothes.

My background is in tailoring and my obsession is with shape and dressing someone to look the best, the sharpest, the slickest and the coolest they can possibly look. Whatever your age or size, style is eternal.

Most importantly clothes should be about having fun and feeling great.

I have also dressed - and more rewardingly – 'real' women with issues not just celebrities! Women with breast cancer and women who are Paralympians with the same energy and love given to each and every person. I have been enriched with amazing stories and experiences and for this I would like to share with you some of my tips.

A BIT OF ADVICE

Gone are the days of mindless spending. Gone are the days of hours spent trawling through shops. As you get older you want to look great but you don't want to spend hours of your day trying to maintain it. I will give you these handy hints to help you achieve this.

IDENTITY AND INFLUENCE

Clothes are part of our identity. I dress for comfort, credibility, power and femininity.

I want to feel effortlessly, elegant and well put together, without being a slave to fashion. Think about where you love to travel and things that make you happy; this is influence.

Tip: Create a mood board. Use Pinterest or pull out pages from fashion magazines and create an actual board of your favourite images.

STYLE

Style is not something you can buy in Bond Street. Style is individual, a feeling and a memory.

I am often asked what keeps us looking good at every age. Simple dressing in clothes that are well cut with structure, beautiful white shirts, soft tailoring, great dresses for day. When you feel good in your clothes that is true style! Buy less and spend well.

Tip: Invest in a stylist, try StitchFix www.stitchfix.co.uk

TAILOR

I advise each season to go into your wardrobe and pull out three pieces that make you happy. Build your key looks around these items as you know these are the pieces that work well. The sense of joy you will have in knowing you have staples that fit you well, will inspire you for the new season style. I know Anthea has a talented Polish lady who tweaks, updates and mends all of her clothes.

Tip: Choose three of your favourite things from your wardrobe, have them made in another fabric and colour by a tailor and invest in a beautiful jacket.

One of my favourite looks I did with Anthea was a white trouser suit, elegant and chic. Anthea rocked the look perfectly, ageless timeless and gorgeous. This is a look that is good at any age.

SHAPE

I love shape. My style icon is Joan Collins. I loved her *Dynasty* wardrobe, for me the shoulders, the belts, the power dressing is everything!

Today I use belts to cinch in waists and play with proportions on coats and dresses.

Tip: Buy a shirt dress (universally flattering), something in a natural fabric. Think about the structure underneath, waist cinching with a belt or with Spanx. Add a shoulder pad to raise the line and narrow the waist.

COLOUR

I have always dressed in black; working in fashion I feel it empowers me. As I get older I love to use colour. Colour enhances your mood, brightens your day makes people feel happy around you.

A great way to use colour is colour blocking. It's extremely flattering to blend red with hot pink but this is not for the faint hearted!

I'm not a fan of the Colour Wheel. If I see one with a client I will often discard it discreetly. Colour should change with your mood and the season.

Tip: Start with a standout bright jacket and wear with cool neutrals, work your way into colour slowly. Add a silk and cashmere scarf in a coordinating pop colour and a bright slick of lipstick. I love Lisou London.

ACCESSORI-ZING!

Jewellery for me is key. It's personal and stylish and can transform the mundane to the extraordinary!

Successful accessorising can be a red lip teamed with a simple outfit and a pair of clip on statement earrings.

This action takes no more than five minutes and can brighten up any outfit and can distract from a multitude of wrinkles.

Tip: Best earrings Vicki Sarge for her one-of-a-kind pieces and Susan Caplan for Vintage and YaYa London.

Always carry a pair of clip on earrings in your bag for an instant day to night look.

REUSE, SUSTAIN

I get to the stage in life where I have a wardrobe filled with clothes but nothing to wear. It's great to pull out the pieces that you love but just don't suit you anymore and perhaps arrange to do some swaps with girlfriends or if you can't bear to eBay get someone to sell it for you.

Create a section of your wardrobe that you can hire out to generate some money through excellent By Rotation or My Wardrobe.

Tip: Rent your wardrobe at By Rotation (all brands) or My Wardrobe HQ (designer). (Boris Johnson's wife Carrie Symonds is said to have hired her wedding dress by Christos Costarellos for just £45 from My Wardrobe HQ.)

SLOW FASHION

I am an advocate of slow fashion, so much so my husband calls me Mr. Bean in my repetitive outfit wearing. Being a creative, I like my focus to be my clients, hence repetition, repetition, repetition in what I know and love. I'm obsessed by fit and cut and I love the feel of natural fabrics. As I get older I try to only wear cotton, linen, silk and cashmere. There are some excellent sustainable options made in small batches and many designers are offering made-to-measure pieces. Again, my philosophy buy less, spend well.

Tip: Pick natural fabrics where possible. Make sure that winter cashmeres and wools are stored correctly. Use mothballs and cloth coverings for winter coats. Dry clean and restore.

Brands: I love Paper London, Anna Mason, Aspiga and Queens of Archive.

HIRE

Hiring is an excellent way of tapping into the high fashion market or current trends without having to spend a fortune on an item you will wear only once. At the moment we have some of the best pieces available on the market to hire, everything from high street to high end and runway looks for all budgets. Balmain, Balenciaga and YSL offer pieces which were once unattainable for mere mortals but they are now within our reach.

Tip: HireStreet www.hirestreet.co.uk (high street to midrange designer).
My Wardrobe HQ www.mywardrobehq.com (designer).
Front Row www.frontrow.uk.com (runway)."

—— **Arabella Boyce** ——

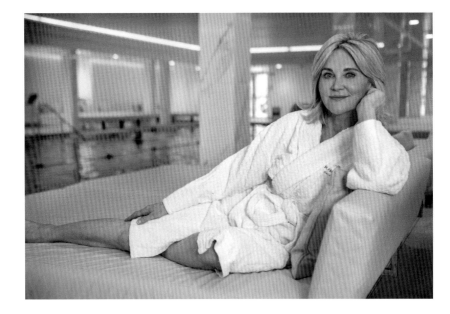

CHAPTER X

— Wellness —

WELLNESS is a word we hear constantly; trawl the internet and you will be bombarded with advice on how to improve wellness. Advertisers love it from elixirs to experiences, whatever they are selling it's going to improve your wellbeing and wellness.

But what do we really need to achieve wellness? We are humans and what separates us from the animals is our intellect and emotion. Looking at my dog Soho asleep beside me I know what makes him healthy and its beautifully simple: he likes to be near to his pack, his purpose in life is to protect us and he shows this by growling at invaders UPS, Royal Mail, and the window cleaner. When he's done something heroic like return from maneuvers outside the encampment he expects a treat and to show me he's ahead of the game and feels safe. Looking at him, I think we all crave a bit of the Soho life!

So, as I advance in my years and gather a little wisdom I have to ask the question, how complicated are we? And the answer is, we're not, it's just the world we live in; a little like our food, it's become over processed and what we are seeking is to become whole again.

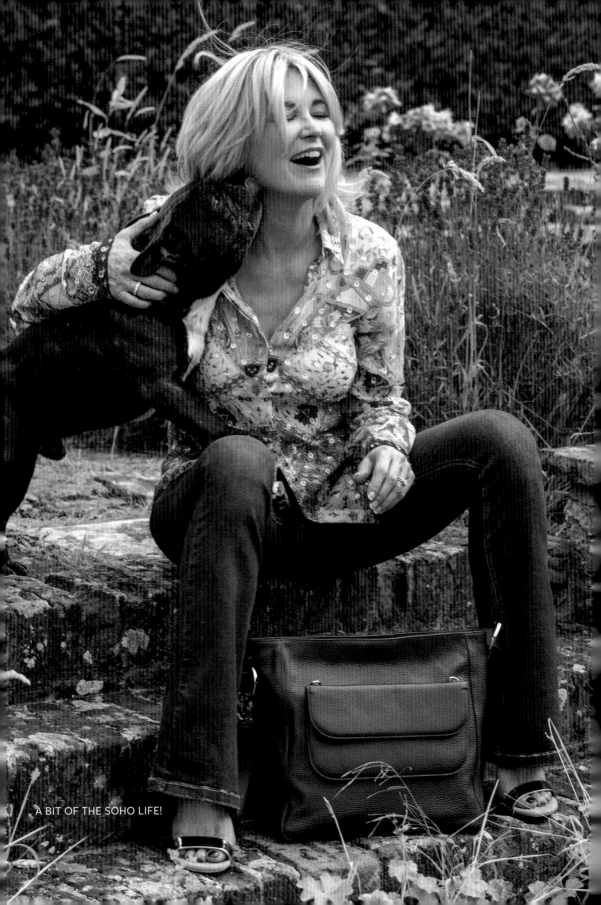

A BIT OF THE SOHO LIFE!

So, where do we start? My advice is with what you can see. Every time I'm in a pickle, I robotically declutter, tidy and clean. I know that doesn't sound like I've handed you the key to wellness but believe me, it works to help clear the mind and feel better about your world. Tackle paperwork, the garage, the shed…even the inside of the car. Don't tell me when you get in a clean car, even the worst journey isn't that little bit better?

Then there's emotional decluttering. Don't hold on to trauma. Divest yourself of bad experiences, do it and do it as quickly as possible. You can't go back so for the sake of the precious years you have on this earth, box it, bury it, learn from it and under no cirumstances return for a rummage around because it will only hold you back.

How I treat my most important asset, the health of my body is a huge part of my wellness. We talk about this in greater depth in the book of course but the key to good health is planted in what you eat and how much you exercise and those things affect your wellness, ie how you feel about yourself.

Another part of my wellness is directly linked to relationships, friends and family. I think as the years go by, friends become family; they protect you, lift you up and of course entertain you. We are primates and interaction is fundamental to our wellness. The recent pandemic put a spotlight on this subject and we saw how isolation is a lethal weapon that attacks the human spirit depleting its resources, making the body ill. It's easy to be lazy; I've done it myself and not made the effort and we often do this when actually we need it most. So, if you are in that hole here's my foot placed across your bum and before I engage power remember the times you've had a night out, or in, with your friends and how enriched you feel in their company.

Finally let's not underestimate the power of a chocolate Hobnob and a cup of Yorkshire tea!!

— *A* —

When I was going through my divorce, wellness certainly didn't appear in my vocabulary. I was heartbroken, distraught and very sad and needed help my lovely friends or family members were not able to provide.

I turned to the wonderful **Donna Robinson**, a holistic therapist and family mediator who'd been recommended to me. She helped me see things in a fresh light and brought positivity back into my life. There's nothing Donna doesn't know about wellness and how important it is to us all.

"EVERYTHING we do in life is connected to our state of mind. For example, someone can say I am going on a diet but if that person is feeling anxious, stressed or worried it is likely they won't succeed due to their mind-set. You have more ability to succeed with determination and positivity in all areas of your life .

I'm fifty-five myself and I recognise how much my life has changed from when I was say in my twenties. As you go through life, your purpose changes. Women in my age group may find they are hormonal. Their children may have flown the nest. They look in the mirror and start to see wrinkles. If you're like me, you're drinking collagen and trying to keep the ageing process at bay. Yet a client of mine who's a lovely lady has let her hair go grey, she's grown tubby and you know what, she couldn't care less. It's about seeing the purpose in the current phase of life and your state of mind. It doesn't matter if you've got the best cream or have had Botox, you're going to glow from within depending on how you're feeling. Unless you've got a positive approach to life, you'll never improve your wellness.

It's all down to your 'Why'. It's like me and my client. I exercise, keep off the pounds and do what I do to make myself feel better. She's happy in her garden and eating more biscuits. I'd say we've each found our own version of wellness. Wellness is about finding your purpose in life. It's about finding positivity in what you do and knowing what you're about. Maintenance is vital too. You need to eat well and exercise to keep your body healthy but true wellness comes from your state of mind which you need to be positive.

I've got a friend who goes round and round in circles. She's only in her forties but always looks completely stressed. She hasn't decided what she wants and what she's doing. Wellness is about knowing what you want in life and why. Everything changes from decade to decade and it's important to note that and actually stop and assess where we are. So many women don't take the time to do that.

In our twenties we're usually looking for a man to have babies with. In our thirties we're running around, dropping them off at school and juggling everything else. In our forties we might be going through a divorce and then the menopause kicks in, the kids have grown up…It's important to note how your life has changed, even for the women who've never married and/or had children. They may be experiencing the death of parents, fewer friends and seeing fewer people. They work a bit more to compensate perhaps. We need to assess every stage of our lives and to decide what makes us happy. And if we discover we're not happy, we have to make changes to achieve wellness.

What is your version of happiness? Is it the Botox? Is it eating well and just taking care of yourself? Is it a holiday every year? What is your happiness? Why do you want your life to be a certain way? What do you want from life? There's no point in going to keep fit classes if you don't enjoy it. Maybe your reason for exercise might be more relaxing like going for a walk on the beach. If you're happy you'll keep doing it.

What makes you happy? Don't worry about other people and what they're doing. What works for you? No two people are the same. I'm a holistic life and wellness coach and when I go and meet people for the first time, I take with me what I call my bag of tools. I use a different tool to help each person because we're all so different with different needs. Don't worry what others are doing. You don't know what's going on in someone else's life and while they might look like their life is perfect, it doesn't mean it is. Your normal is not necessarily someone else's. Social media places a lot of pressure on us. The millions of websites extolling the virtues of the latest neck cream for instance. You see all these adverts for baggy arms or injections for getting rid of wrinkles on your hands. Have them by all means if it's going to make you feel better about yourself but truly, you can only achieve wellness from within".

—— **Donna Robinson** ——

SLEEP

As with all people who do shift work or perform their job at what we'd refer to as 'unsociable hours' after joining *GMTV* in my thirties, I became obsessed by sleep.

To perform at your optimum level and not look tired you need sleep, but not any old sleep, it must be good sleep, the right amount, at the right time.

Everyone is different in their approach but for me who's not a napper the only way I could tackle this was to completely time shift my life. Bedtime 9pm, alarm 4am. This worked well apart from Monday morning when I'd slipped into normality over the weekend and if I was tempted by an irresistible offer of a midweek night out.

It didn't take long for me to realise that lack of sleep not only left me looking less than my best (you need your beauty sleep', is actually true) but I couldn't function at my best. A decent night's sleep is vital to our wellness, yet so many of us don't make sleep a top priority.

Health coach **Ailsa Hichens** (see also Chapter III Nutrition) is an expert when it comes to the link between sleep and wellness and here offers us the benefit of her expertise:

"GETTING a decent night's sleep is a real game changer in the world of wellness. When you have a terrible night's sleep you really know about it. Think back to a time you had a run of good sleep. You were probably walking around with a spring in your step, more focussed and intentional about everything you were doing. Now cast your mind to a time when you had a truly terrible night's sleep. Apart from feeling like you were dragging yourself through the day, everything felt hard, right? And everyone got on your nerves. Your temper was short, you made terrible food choices (you needed the energy) and the experience of being you that day was not the best, to say the least.

Sleep comes into the same kind of category as drinking water. Do more of it, your body and health would thank you for it. Both are free. You could sleep more or drink more water at any time.

Your sleep is made up of a series of stages that repeat in cycles through the night. The length of each stage might vary as you go through the night but, broadly, each cycle is made up like this:

- **Stage one** is the lightest sleep. Your body isn't fully relaxed although brain activity has started to slow. You can be easily woken. Think 'catnap.' If you're not disturbed, you'll move into the next sleep stage.

- **Stage two** is also fairly light. Your muscles relax, your breathing slows, as does your heart rate. Body temperature also lowers. Think 'powernap'.

- **Stage three** is deeper sleep. In fact, it's actually called 'deep sleep' and is the most restorative sleep of all. It dictates how well your body repairs and protects itself. Skimp on this and you won't feel fully refreshed. If you're woken in this phase, you'll likely feel a bit befuddled for a few minutes while you adjust.

- **Stage four** is called REM sleep. REM stands for Rapid Eye Movement and, in this phase of sleep, your eyes do literally dart about while most of your muscles are temporarily paralysed. It's the sleep phase in which you are most likely to dream, and it's important for learning, creativity, memory, and mood.

There's an important relationship between sleep and your mental health. The two are intertwined and the symptoms of lack of sleep and poor mental health are very similar. And, if you struggle with anxiety or depression, you'll find it harder to sleep, while lack of sleep can exacerbate symptoms of both. It's a horrible, horrible cycle.

Lack of sleep on a regular basis also increases your risk of cancer, including aggressive breast cancer. Don't shoot the messenger. Not only that, the chances of getting heart disease, type 2 diabetes or metabolic syndrome also shoot up.
Most of my clients are women in their forties and beyond, and one of the things that bothers them most about their health is weight gain, and specifically the kind that doesn't seem to shift no matter what you try. There are several ways that sleep impacts on this.

It's an acknowledged fact that people who sleep less tend to weigh more than those who get a good night's sleep.

Lack of sleep increases levels of the stress hormone cortisol. Here's why that matters. In some ways, we haven't really evolved that much since cavewoman times when stress hormones had a really functional benefit. An increase in these hormones primed you for having the energy, tenacity, and agility to run away from the saber-toothed tiger. Energy (aka fat) would be stored in the easiest place for it to be used in times of need – your middle. That may have worked in prehistoric times, but this strategy just leads to a muffin top these days since we rarely need to run away from the source of stress.

Stress also destabilises your blood sugar levels, leading to cravings, which are never for the healthiest foods.

Lack of sleep also messes with the release of appetite-controlling hormones ghrelin (the hunger hormone) and leptin (the one that tells your body you're full). And not in a favourable way. You feel hungrier and your satiety hormones are broken, so it's easy to overeat.

Lack of zzzzz also leads to changes in the reward centre of the brain. You literally think about food differently. You don't need the science to tell you (although it does), that the foods you're most drawn to under these circumstances are those most likely to see the scale move north.

I think that's decided then? Simply put, if you want to be healthier and happier, if you want to achieve wellness, you need to take the business of sleep seriously.

HOW TO SLEEP BETTER

- Keep your blood sugar levels steady through the day. Base your meals on plenty of protein, lots of vegetables and a limited amount of starchy foods such as bread, rice and potatoes. This stops your blood sugars from spiking then dropping too low at night and waking you up.

- Create yourself a caffeine curfew. The half-life of caffeine is between five and eight hours, so you want to give yourself enough time to get all of it out of your system by the time you hit the pillow. Basically, cut out or cut down on tea and coffee after 4pm.

- The same goes for alcohol. It disturbs the sleep-wake cycle. It's better not to drink a few hours before bed if you want your REM sleep to be intact.

- Getting outdoors is IT if you want to sleep well. Being outdoors in the sunshine (or even using light therapy in winter months) is known to lift levels of the 'happy hormone' serotonin, which is the warm-up act to melatonin.

- Exercise is generally regarded as one of the very best things you can do for every single aspect of your health. If your schedule allows, exercising in the morning is best and, for rigorous exercise like HIIT, spinning, running and so on, try not to work out after 4ish.

- Screens kill your sleep. Switch off the TV, phone and tablet at least ninety minutes before bed. In fact, it might be a good idea to banish tech from the bedroom altogether.

- Consider room temperature. Even if you're a person who likes to stay warm, the best temperature for your room is between 15°C and 18°C.

- People always say sleep in a blacked-out room. It works. If you can do that, great. If your room isn't dark and – understandably, you're not sure you want to fork out on blackout curtains – try a silk sleep mask. Silk masks are kind to ageing skin and are very comfortable to wear.

- I'm often asked what I think of supplements and my personal view is that they bridge the gap between an OK diet and a great one. For a good night's sleep, look at a high-quality multi-vitamin that uses the most absorbable forms of **B vitamins** and **magnesium**. Magnesium is a wonder mineral, which is helpful for all kinds of things, including stress, lady hormones and sleep. For anything to do with hormones or mood, I like a high-strength omega 3 supplement. Finally, you can't just buy yourself melatonin in the UK as you can in the US, but you can buy the next best thing, Montmorency cherry. This is a very tart cherry with naturally high levels of melatonin".

—— **Ailsa Hichens** ——

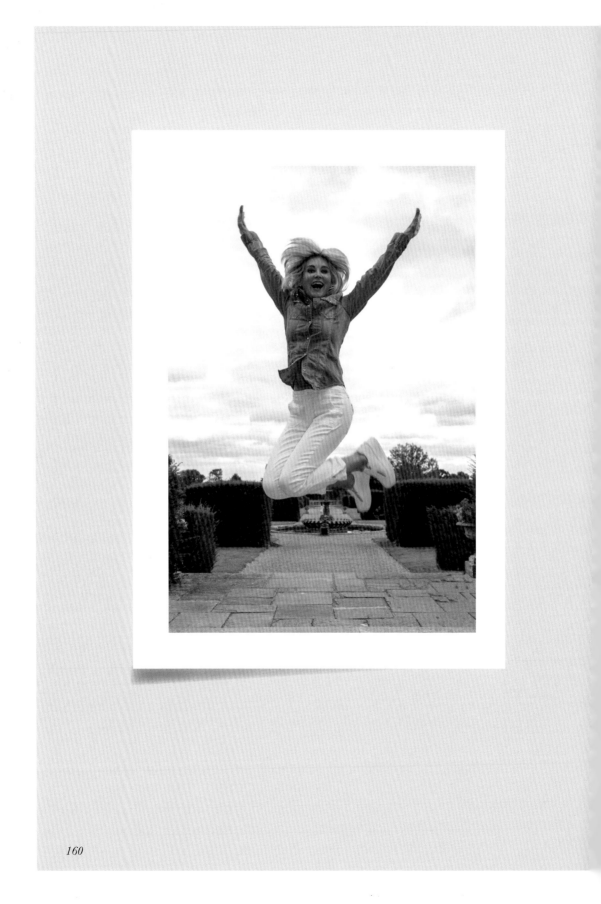

THANKS

— to Our Expert Contributors —

Mr Nick Panay BSc MBBS FRCOG MFSRH
Consultant Gynaecologist, Subspecialist in Reproductive Medicine, Queen Charlotte's & Chelsea Hospital and Chelsea & Westminster Hospital London. Professor of Practice, Imperial College London. Founder and Director of the International Centre for Hormone Health. Medical Advisory Council member and past Chair of the British Menopause Society (BMS). President Elect of the International Menopause Society (IMS). Past Editor-in-Chief of Climacteric (The Journal of the IMS). Council Member and Past Director of Conferences, RCOG.
www.hormonehealth.co.uk

Dr Clare Spencer MA (Cantab) MB BChir DM MRCOG MRCGP
Registered menopause specialist, GP partner and co-founder My Menopause Centre. A busy doctor, Dr Spencer runs both NHS and private menopause services. She has a passion for educating women and doctors about the menopause transition and has delivered numerous talks to both. She has both written and contributed to publications and books on women's health including authoring the Non Menstrual Vaginal Bleeding chapter in *Women's Health in Primary Care* by Anne Connolly and Amanda Britton.
www.mymenopausecentre.com

Helen Normoyle Co-Founder My Menopause Centre
Women's wellbeing warrior on a mission to raise awareness of the menopause to help empower women with the knowledge they need to embrace this new chapter – and thrive.
www.mymenopausecentre.com

Paula Kerr Founder and Owner Fitter Stronger
Author *Fitter Stronger – Resilience – If You're Going Through Hell, Keep Going*. Fitter Stronger offers classes, personal training, wellness breaks in the UK and South Africa, NHS and private medicine rehab clinics and a youth fitness and motivation programme for primary, secondary and further education.
www.fitterstronger.org
Instagram: @fitter.stronger

Regina Kerschbaumer Founder Yoga Orchid and Yoga Orchid Yinstitute
Author *Yoga, Coffee and a Glass of Wine: A Yoga Journey*.
Trained with Yin Yoga Master Paul Grilley in the USA (120hrs RYT).
www.yogaorchid.com
Instagram: @yogaorchid_regina

Duncan Knowles Assistant to the Director of Training,
The Constructive Teaching Centre Registered Alexander Technique Coach. Actor, voice teacher and coach.
www.constructiveteachingcentre.com
Telephone: +44 020 7727 7222

Lorraine Nicolle MSc, PGCert, BA (Hons), Dip BCNH
Registered Nutritionist (MBANT), Nutritional Therapist (CNHC) and Nutrition Educator (PG Cert). Author *Biochemical Imbalances in Disease*, *The Functional Nutrition Cookbook* and *Eat to Get Younger*.
www.lorrainenicollenutrition.co.uk

Ailsa Hichens
Nutritional Therapist (BANT) and Health Coach (CNHC)
www.foodfabulous.co.uk
Instagram: @foodfabulousnutrition

Lino Carbosiero MBE
Awarded MBE for Services to Hairdressing in 2014. Works at Daniel Galvin Salon.
www.danielgalvin.com
Instagram: @linocarbosiero

Wendy Nixon Owner Armstrong Cuthbert Salon
Over thirty-five years of industry experience. Qualifications with Sassoon, Aveda, Wella and Fantastic Hairdresser. Voted London's leading hair salon in 2016.
www.armstrongcuthbert.co.uk
Instagram: @armstrongcuthbert

Anabel Kingsley Brand President and Consultant Trichologist Philip Kingsley
www.philipkingsley.com
Instagram: @anabel_kingsley

Dr Emma Wedgeworth MA MBBS MRCP UK (Derm) DCH
Consultant Dermatologist & Skincare Expert.
www.dremmawedgeworth.com
Instagram: @dremwedgeworth

Helen Hand Makeup Artist
Works for ITV. Makeup artist on *Lorraine*. Has made up every living Prime Minister.
www.helenhandmakeup.com
Instagram: @helenhandmakeup

Grace Fodor Founder and Director Studio10 Makeup
www.studio10beauty.com
Instagram: @studio10makeup

Dr Andrew Weber MB.BS, DRCOG MemberBCAM – British College of Aesthetic Medicine, FRSM – Fellow of The Royal Society of Medicine, FPCert – Family Planning Certificate, LOC (IUD/IUS) – Letter of Competence, Member FSRH – Faculty of Sexual and Reproductive Health, Member BMS – British Menopause Society.
www.bodyvie.com

Fiona Sellars RGN Bsc (Hons) PGDip
Independent Nurse Prescriber.
Director and lead clinician at Surrey Hills
Skin Clinic.
Fiona@surreyhillsskinclinic.co.uk
Instagram: @SHSkinClinic

Dr Kunal Patel MUDr Prague 2010
Founder Love Teeth Dental, UK's first
clinic to achieve Invisalign Diamond
accreditation within a year.
Senior Master with Fast Braces.
Dental Phobia Certified.
www.drkp.dentist or
www.loveteethdental.co.uk

Ali Mearza MB BS FRCOphth
Consultant Ophthalmic Surgeon and
Director OCL Vision.
www.oclvision.com

Arabella Boyce Stylist
Fashion stylist and Editor.
Red carpet.
Instagram: @arabellaboycestylist

Donna Robinson Holistic Therapist
and Family Mediator
wellbeingforyou1@gmail.com
www.wellbeingforyou.org.uk

Alison Webster Photographer
www.Alison@alisonwebster.co.uk
Instagram: @alisonvwebster

INDEX